Shepherdess

Shepherdess

NOTES

FROM

THE

FIELD

Joan Jarvis Ellison

Purdue University Press
West Lafayette, Indiana

99 98 97 96   5 4 3

The paper used in this book meets the minimum requirements of American National Standard for Information Sciences—Permanence of Paper for Printed Library Materials, ANSI Z39.48-1984.

Printed in the United States of America

Photograph on page 116 by Mel Zierke
Design by Chiquita Babb

LIBRARY OF CONGRESS CATALOGING-IN-PUBLICATION DATA

Ellison, Joan Jarvis, 1948–
    Shepherdess : notes from the field / Joan Jarvis Ellison.
        p.   cm.
    ISBN 1-55753-070-X (alk. paper)
        1. Ellison, Joan Jarvis, 1948– . 2. Women shepherds—Minnesota—
Pelican Rapids—Biography. 3. Farm life—Minnesota—Pelican Rapids. I. Title
    SF375.32.E45A3 1995
    636.3'01'092—dc20   95-4199
    [B]   CIP

Contents

Shepherdess

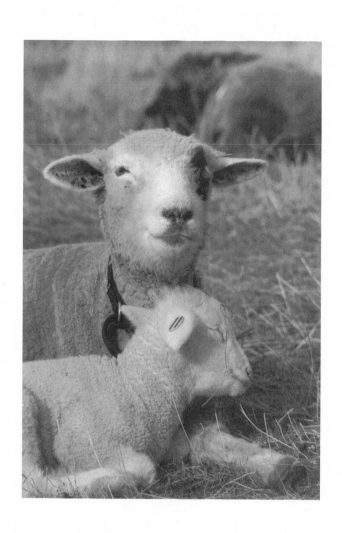

An Introduction

One June I bought four sheep as pets. The following March, I began to be a shepherdess.

The entire process actually began years before, when Amber, my first daughter, was born. I retired as a biochemist, the career for which I had trained and which I enjoyed, to become a full-time mother. However, after ten years of being a nonperson in many social situations because of this career choice, I was ready for a change. I needed to be an authority on something. I needed to feel as if I could once again pay my own way, both monetarily and philosophically.

I had grown weary of being introduced as Dr. Ellison's wife, Joan, or as Amber and Laurel's mom. I had quietly listened too many times while physicians and their nurse wives discussed medicine around me. I didn't like being invited to be on committees because I was the doctor's wife. No one listens to mothers, not even their own children. I needed to be a professional again, an expert, in charge.

There were no jobs requiring a master's degree in biochemistry in our rural community of 1,865 people. I wasn't willing to give up all mothering and drive two hours a day to do biochemistry nine hours a day in the nearest town with a university. Besides, biochemistry had changed a lot in the ten years I had been a mother. I was no longer proficient.

I had no training for the high-level careers that did exist close to home, such as nursing or teaching. My interest in assembly-line work or clerking was as non-existent as jobs in biochemistry.

What I needed was a new career—one that I could pursue at home, without the two-hour drive to a university. I enjoyed knitting mittens, hats, scarves, and sweaters, turning long, beautifully colored strands of yarn into clothing. I was learning to spin on the spinning wheel my folks had bought me, converting clouds of carded wool into regular, finely twisted yarn. I enjoyed the feel of the wool and the feeling of accomplishment when I finished a project, from raw wool to warm mittens. I loved animals. At the time, we had one parakeet, two dogs, three cats, and twenty-five brown New Hampshire chickens. We lived in the country, where people raised cows and sheep. Sheep were small, I would be able to handle them easily. I would become a shepherdess, and my projects would really be mine from beginning to end, from sheep to sweater.

As a shepherdess, I would be a member of a small but respected profession. I would make my own decisions, and the sheep would mind me—a habit my children were rapidly outgrowing. I would be earning real money. And when people asked me, "What do you do?" I could answer with pride. Of course, I would also have to work hard, but that didn't occur to me immediately. I blithely went ahead and bought the sheep after Laurel's first year at school.

All summer, the four sheep I purchased in June wandered picturesquely around our pastures, keeping the grasses and apple trees well trimmed. Laurel, Amber, Dave, and I visited them daily. They were soon eating out of our hands.

"I can handle this," I thought. "Maybe some lambs would be nice." So in October we bred our sheep to a big ornery ram who lived in a neighboring county.

Almost immediately, things got harder. First, snow covered the pasture grasses. With the grass unavailable for food, I had to fork twenty pounds of hay over the fence every day. Next year, with eight sheep, it would be forty pounds. I began to have second thoughts about lambing. But it was too late for second thoughts: my sheep were all irreversibly pregnant.

With time, I got stronger and feeding got easier. I persuaded myself that fifty pounds wasn't so heavy. Then the temperature plummeted. The water in my beautifully insulated and electrically heated water tank froze overnight. I filled a bucket with water at the pump, pulled the pasture gate open as far as possible against the snow bank (about eight inches) and squeezed myself through, holding the four-gallon bucket over my head. The water that splashed out of the bucket froze on contact with my jacket and jeans. It took slightly longer to freeze in my hair. I waded through two-foot drifts in the first pasture, hugging the bucket to my chest. I climbed the fence, turned the corner, and waded through more drifts to the winter pasture. "Next year," I thought, "we'll build a gate right into the winter pasture."

The water left in my bucket filled the trough barely one-fourth full. I began my journey back to the pump. By the time I squeezed out through the gate, I decided that the sheep could wait until noon for their second bucket of water. By noon, the water in the trough was frozen again. I made three trips with water that day.

3

During the night it snowed again. The next morning I couldn't budge the gate. It was snowed shut for the rest of the winter.

Out of desperation, I decided to believe what I'd read in one of my sheep books: "Sheep would rather eat snow than drink water." None of the other books had mentioned it, but I was out of ideas. My sheep would have to eat snow. Fortunately, there was no shortage.

I muddled through January and February, reading and rereading my sheep books. Lambing season was rapidly approaching. I was not ready. Every book had lists of necessary lambing supplies, and every list was different. After I read beyond towels, iodine, twine, hair dryer (hair dryer?), the words became unpronounceable and, as far as I was concerned, completely unfamiliar. What in God's name was an oxytetracycline uterine bolus, and where could I find one? Should I ask at the veterinary, the feed elevator, or the farm-supply store?

My ignorance was overwhelming me. What good is a prestigious, unusual, respected job if everyone can tell you are a fool? I wanted a job at which I could excel, at which I could be the expert. Instead, I had entered a field in which I found myself ignorant of even the simplest things. Admitting ignorance, although necessary at times, was painful, and I wanted to avoid it if at all possible.

I found almost everything on my lambing lists at the farm-supply store. And I found it myself without showing my ignorance to the store clerks. But I still didn't know how to use my supplies. Finally I wrote out a list of questions (just like when I had had an appointment with my obstetrician) and called one of the local vets. Dr. Magnusson was young and businesslike but very helpful. He talked fast and had a lot to say. I wrote down about one third of it. Statements such as "You probably

won't need the uterine boluses with such a small flock"
were comforting but not enough. What if I did need
them? Would I have time to drive thirty miles each way
to buy them, or did they have to be inserted immediately? (I had learned something, anyway: uterine boluses
have to be inserted—in uteruses.)

I finished lambing preparations on the first day my
sheep could possibly lamb. Any time in the next six
weeks, four baby lambs would be born. I was uncertain
and afraid. No question, I was in over my head. I never
should have bred those sheep. The books were not
encouraging. They listed and then illustrated eight common lambing problems. Then they told what to do for
each problem. The instructions read something like this:
(1) determine the problem; (2) wash your hands and
arm with soap and warm water; (3) lubricate your hand
and arm; (4) don't panic. Honestly, every single book
had point number four listed. That's like telling someone
not to think about purple elephants. Besides, I had panicked way back at point two, when it said to wash your
hands and arm. Arm!

It got worse from there. Next the books said to
reach into the ewe's uterus to find the missing part of the
lamb's body and to ease it out. Reach into the ewe's
uterus? Five years ago I had trouble cutting up a chicken
for dinner. Now I'm supposed to reach into a ewe's
uterus!

Finally, the day I'd been dreading arrived. One of
the ewes lay down on the floor of the tiny old feed shed
we were using for lambing and started to grunt. I
checked her in half an hour. Still lying there, still grunting. It was happening! And of course it was happening
when Dave was at work and the kids were asleep.

I called my friend Jan, who lived an hour's drive

away. "Hurry!" I said. "All the books say labor lasts an hour. And it's been half an hour since she lay down."

"I'm coming," said Jan. "Don't panic!"

"Don't panic!" I thought as I hustled around the house collecting towels, sharp knife, soap, reference book, and a bucket of warm water. "Don't panic. Don't panic. Don't panic!" I forced myself to sit quietly in the kitchen and reread the chapter on lambing. Then, not at all reassured, I gathered my bundles and walked slowly out to the lambing shed.

All four ewes were lying on the straw-covered floor grunting. Panic!

Fortunately, Jan arrived. "What's happening?" she asked.

"I don't know." I rushed her out of the car, over the fence, across the frozen pasture, and into the partial warmth of the dimly lit shed. "They can't all be in labor at the same time. But they are all lying on the floor grunting."

"Why can't they all be in labor?" she asked, examining the slightly grubby straw carefully before sitting down on it.

"They can't because I need to learn about lambing one at a time, not four at a time." Tight control kept me from shouting, but my voice was still overly loud and cracked when I spoke. "Do you want to read the chapter on lambing?"

"Yeah, I guess that would be a good idea."

While Jan read about the problems of lambing, I stared at Polar Bear, the ewe who had lain down first. Her brown eyes were wide and staring. Her white belly was distended. I saw a ripple. "There!" I shouted, startling four ewes and two people. "Was that a contraction?"

Jan looked up from the book. "I didn't see it. Did it look like when you were in labor?"

"I didn't see myself when I was in labor. I didn't even know I was in labor. I just thought I had stomach cramps. If I couldn't tell on myself, how can I tell on a sheep?"

"What time is it?" Jan asked.

"Eleven-thirty. She's been in labor for two and a half hours. Maybe I should call the vet." My voice was reluctant. Calling the vet meant definitely displaying my ignorance to someone other than an equally ignorant friend.

"Let's watch for a while longer," Jan said. "Do you think you'll remember what to do for all the lamb mispresentations?"

"You mean if they don't come out nose and front feet first?"

Jan nodded.

"Never! That's what you're here for, to read the directions to me. All I remember is not to tie a rope around the lamb's neck."

Jan opened the book to look at an illustration. "It says one leg and nose forward is the second most common way for lambs to be born. Do you remember what to do for that?"

"Something about reaching in and following the one leg across the chest to the other leg, tying a rope around it and pulling it out."

"You're right." She read a little more. "It also says to be sure to keep your hand on the lamb so you don't accidentally break the umbilical cord."

I thought seriously about what we were doing, sitting in a little shed in the middle of a cold winter night waiting to help a ewe give birth to a lamb. It was terrifying! "Jan, I'll never be able to stick my hand in there! What will I do if two feet and a nose don't come out first? I'm so afraid the ewe will die or the lamb will die. I don't think I could stand it if one died and it was my fault." I looked at Polar Bear again. Nothing was happening.

"What if the lamb is breech and nothing is happening because she's is too tired to try any more?"

My heart was pounding. My stomach was tied in knots. My belly muscles felt like they had been tight for days. I couldn't stand the waiting. I couldn't tolerate not knowing what to do.

Jan laid her hand on my arm. "Let's compare her to the other ewes."

"Okay, you watch Cocoa—she's the other white one. I'll watch Fair and Brownie."

We sat for a long time, listening to the moan of the wind outside the shed and the quiet grunting of the sheep inside. As I watched I began to relax. They seemed so at peace that I almost had to be. My attention was divided among three sheep, one white and two dark, trying to see any differences in their behavior. They were different in many ways. Fair had huge black ears that stuck out; she lay closest to me, completely unafraid. Brownie was a warm, beautiful brown color and had delicate features. Even in the security of the shed, she lay backed into a corner, as far away from us as possible. Polar Bear had a cluster of curls in the middle of her broad forehead and a small black nose. She, too, disliked people and watched us warily.

They chewed and grunted and lay there.

Jan spoke. "Cocoa is eating my shoelace."

"Well, that doesn't sound like she's in much distress. I think Fair's going to sleep—she just laid her head on my foot. They're all acting the same. Polar Bear and Brownie aren't as relaxed as Fair and Cocoa, but now that I think of it, they're always that way." This was becoming anticlimactic.

"Have you seen any more contractions?" Jan asked.

"No. In fact, I've almost decided she was just taking a deep breath."

"What about the grunting?" Jan persisted. She had driven a long way on a cold night to see a lamb being born.

"I've realized," I said, "that they always make grunting noises. And they all seem to be chewing their cud."

Jan and I looked at each other and smiled ruefully. "Let's go in and make some hot chocolate. I'm getting awfully cold."

We left the light and odor and relative warmth of the barn and walked across the cold, dark pasture. A wind blew fresh from the southwest. The stars glittered icily in the sky. I felt good. The panic was gone. I knew the sheep better. It hardly mattered that no lamb had been born. We warmed our insides with hot chocolate and our outsides in front of the woodstove. At 4:30 A.M. we pulled on our jackets, hats, and mittens and trudged out to the lambing shed again. All four ewes were sleeping. Jan and I went back to the house, curled up in front of the fire, and fell asleep ourselves.

Two weeks later, Polar Bear had two healthy, energetic white lambs, all by herself. Then Cocoa had a little brown ewe lamb, Brownie had a black ewe, and Fair had a huge black ram—all by themselves. No washed hands, no lubricated arms, no panic. After all, shepherdesses don't panic.

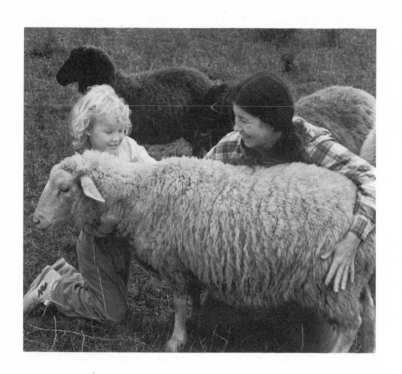

Sheep Don't Bite

Both the sheep and I had survived lambing. Amber and Laurel immediately named the new baby lambs: Cinnamon, Puddles, Persephone, and Charlie. We didn't name the ram lamb because he was scheduled for our freezer in the fall. Not that a number instead of a name keeps you from getting attached to an animal. We knew it would be hard for all of us when slaughter time came around.

The lambs raced joyously around the pasture, playing king of the mountain on their mothers' backs, and quickly learned to cluster around humans, butting and baaing for corn.

Watching lambs brought smiles to faces. I melted inside when I held one cradled in my arms, rubbing my cheek across its fuzzy, bony little head. The girls spent hours in the pasture just holding the lambs. Even Dave, the reserved member of the family, couldn't resist them.

In June, with five lambs enlivening our days, the decision to have more sheep came easily. And this time I'd buy my own ram; then we'd be sure of a new crop of lambs next spring. I was fairly self-confident when I set out to buy the ram.

BUT I STILL remembered the humiliation of my first two sheep buying trips, which had managed to destroy whatever self-esteem I had developed in my professional and family life. Before that, the closest I had been to buying sheep was buying groceries, and I had the distinct feeling that the two activities were pretty unrelated. When I bought groceries, I went to the supermarket with my careful list of the dairy products, meat, fruit, vegetables, and bread I needed. Everything was neatly arranged on shelves and lighted to enhance its desirability. I strolled up and down the aisles to the strains of Muzak. I made my selections by habit, impulse, or by careful reading of the labels. The colors of the fruits and vegetables, the bright packaging, and the enticing aromas from the bakery section all made shopping pleasant.

Buying lamb chops had certainly not prepared me for buying sheep. On my first sheep shopping trip, I was led into a dark, smelly, noisy barn. Cobwebbed posts receded into the gloom. Light from a small window, far away, filtered through the dust in the air. Lambs milled around us, baaaing enthusiastically for a treat. The noise was incredible! Every lamb had her mouth open. They all sounded angry, or at least irritated with our slowness.

Wendy, the shepherdess, gave me a handful of corn.

"If you like the looks of a ewe," she shouted, "offer her some corn. When she starts eating, grab her."

Again, no past experience had prepared me for this. Even when I selected live lobsters at the fish market, I didn't have to stick my hand in the tank as bait.

I had never touched a sheep before, only seen them at the state fair. Now I hesitantly held a handful of corn toward a big, black, floppy-eared ewe. She immediately nuzzled my hand. "Oh!" I jumped away, shocked by the feel of her mouth.

"They don't bite," Wendy laughed. "They pick up the corn with their lips."

Somewhat reassured, I held out my hand again. Floppy ears came back for another taste of corn. I reached slowly for the wool on her shoulders, grabbed tightly, and hollered, "I've got one."

Floppy ears headed for the far side of the barn with me running alongside. The lobster in the tank flashed through my head—at least this ewe didn't have claws. Suddenly she darted around a corner and left me plastered against a post, nursing a bruised shoulder.

"Did you like the way her wool felt?" Wendy asked, laughing. "Next time, grab a leg. Then she can't run as well."

Wendy was dressed in ragged blue jeans, old tennis shoes, and a faded blue sweatshirt. I looked down at my new jeans, clogs, and designer T-shirt, my naive idea of how a shepherdess dressed. Oh well, they were washable.

I enticed a brown ewe to my side with another handful of corn.

"How does she look?" asked Wendy from directly behind me.

"Okay, I guess." I really didn't know what I wanted. A nice fleece was my main criterion. I thought I knew how to judge fleeces. Obviously, clean fleeces were superior to fleeces full of hay and manure, and brown fleeces spun up into pretty brown yarn. Basically, I spun whatever wool my fiber store sold.

"Let's look at her." Wendy grabbed a hind leg and held on. The ewe struggled. I knelt down in the manure and put my arms around the ewe's neck. Then Wendy straddled her back.

"See how long the fleece is?" she said. "That will be easy to spin. Do you like the color?"

13

"Yes. And I like the little waves in her hair," I said.

Wendy laughed again. "Wool. Sheep have wool, not hair. The little waves in the wool are called crimp. You're right, though. They are nice."

My ignorance was obvious. No amount of past education or experience could help me out here. I couldn't even touch a sheep without showing my ignorance. But damned if I was going to continue to sound dumb.

"I like this one and that floppy-eared one," I said. "That'll give me a black one and a brown one. That's enough to start with."

After we loaded the sheep into the pickup truck, we tied two-by-fours and baling twine across any possible escape route. Amber and Laurel gazed out of the window, entranced. As we pulled out of the barnyard, Amber said, "I want the brown one. Her name is Brownie."

"I want a white one," Laurel said.

"You'll have to wait," I said. "We'll give the black one to your cousin Jared. He wants to call her Fair."

MY NEXT VENTURE in sheep shopping, that same summer, was similar to the first, except all the sheep in Barry's barn looked alike: small, woolly, and white. The smell was incredible. Incredibly bad. The source of the smell was readily apparent. Sheep droppings covered the barn floor, old and new sheep droppings. The hundreds of lambs crowded body to body into the barn had been very busy.

Barry, the shepherd, pulled on his boots and led me through the sea of sheep, shoving them out of our way with his knees as he walked. "You should have worn boots instead of running shoes," he said.

"I don't have any. But it's okay if these shoes get dirty."

"You'll have to get boots. Everything gets caught in

the soles of tennis shoes. You don't want to take this smell everywhere you go."

When we were somewhere in the middle of that baaing, pushing, defecating ocean, Barry handed me a fat orange crayon and walked away.

"Use this crayon to mark the sheep you're interested in," he said. "Then I'll look them up in the book."

I hurriedly made a broad orange streak down the noses of the four unremarkable white sheep standing next to me.

"Okay," I said.

Barry had settled under a glowing light bulb. He looked up from his book. "Done already? Fine. Read me the numbers on their ear tags, and I'll tell you about their parents."

The numbers were on little silver strips. The light from the barn door didn't quite reach our corner. I had to put my nose right against the lamb's face to read her ear tag.

"Number 464," I read.

"She's a twin out of Solomon and Maggie. Solomon is a Lincoln-Finn cross, and Maggie is Montadale."

I grasped at the one word that made any sense to me. "Twin!" One baby at a time seemed more than enough. "Does that mean she'll have twins too?"

"Yeah." Barry grinned. "The more twins you have, the more money you earn," he said. "That's why I'm using a Lincoln-Finn ram. Finn sheep usually have multiple births."

Maybe buying sheep was like buying groceries, after all. The shepherd's records were like the contents label on a loaf of bread: flour, water, yeast. Number 464 had a contents label, too: Montadale, Lincoln, Finn. As long as I knew the meaning of the words, I was fine. I now had a partial meaning for the word "Finn"—twins. It wasn't until much later that I learned Finn meant many things: twins; light, fine fleeces; good mothers; and slow growth.

I gathered my courage. "Tell me about Lincoln and Montadale sheep," I said.

"The people I bought Solomon from sell their fleeces to handspinners," Barry said. "But I don't know what it is about Lincoln fleeces that is good for handspinners."

"The long wool is easy to spin," I said, echoing Wendy. I was learning.

"Montadale sheep have nice open faces," Barry said. "That way you don't have to shear their faces or worry about eye infections."

In my head I filed "open faced." Number 464 had no long wool on her face—perhaps that was what "open faced" meant.

"Pick another number," he said.

"1080."

"1080 is Corriedale, North Country Cheviot, Lincoln, Finn, and Suffolk."

I nodded blankly.

"Corriedales and Suffolks gain weight well," he added.

I realized that hearing the genealogies of more sheep, though educational, was not going to help me make a decision at this point. I didn't know what I wanted. Two white ewes had been the extent of my planning.

"I'll take 464 and 1080," I said. I felt like I had just bought two different brands of white bread. I couldn't see the differences. But according to the labels, they were different.

Laurel watched as we loaded 464 and 1080 into the pickup. "I want the one with the pink nose," she said. "Her name is Cocoa."

I looked at the sheep in surprise. I hadn't seen any

differences except the numbers on their tags. Sure enough, Cocoa had a fat pink nose and a big head. The other sheep had a fine-featured face with a small black nose.

"Zach wants to call his sheep Polar Bear," Laurel said after we climbed into the pickup.

"They're already named," I said to Barry as he opened the gate for us. "Cocoa and Polar Bear."

He laughed. His sheep had names, too. Barry waved as we drove through the gate. "Good luck, shepherdess."

THAT HAD BEEN the first year. In the meantime, I had done a lot more reading and talked to a lot of shepherds. I was no longer afraid of sheep who had twins. I wanted more Finn in my flock. I had carefully examined and spun the fleeces shorn from my four ewes. The fibers in my four fleeces ranged from medium to coarse. They would not spin up into a soft, wearable yarn. I needed a ram with a soft, fine fleece to cross with my Lincoln-Finn sheep. The Targee rams bred at the agricultural research station north of us seemed the perfect answer.

I knew that I wanted a Targee-Finn cross. Finn for the twins and triplets. Targee for the fine, crimpy, heavy fleeces. I had come a long way in a year. I had also found a shepherdess mentor, Edith. We were buying the ram together.

When we arrived at the agricultural research station, the shepherd was in his office. He was dressed in a suit and tie and sitting at a desk. Edith and I were wearing our barn boots, grubby jeans, and ragged T-shirts. The shepherd called his assistant, who walked with us across the campus to a sunny, open building containing a dozen new-looking paddocks with three to six sheep in each paddock. Three rams were penned in the last paddock, waiting for us.

Edith looked at the first ram critically. "This one is kind of knock-kneed."

"All right. Cross him off the list." The shepherd's assistant easily caught a second ram for us to look at. We felt his fleece, looked at his head and legs.

"He looks pretty good," said Edith.

"I think so, too," I agreed. "His face is open, and I like this dense, crimpy fleece. It's perfect for crossing with our long-wooled sheep." In an undertone I added, "One of my books said we should feel their testicles."

"Like pears at the supermarket?" Edith laughed. "You can squeeze his balls if you want to, but I don't think I'll try it."

Blushing furiously, I asked the shepherd to hold the ram tightly. Then I squatted beside the lamb, pulled his body against my chest, and tentatively touched his scrotum. He certainly had one. But that was all the information I could get from touching it. The book hadn't told me what to feel for.

We paid for ram number 2 and loaded him into his own traveling crate. I had worn boots but hadn't gotten them dirty. Even so, the pungent odor of ram enveloped us all the way home.

I HAD PURCHASED my two colored sheep on looks, just as I'd buy lobsters. I used the list of ingredients to select my two white ones, like choosing bread. And I had tried to test the testicles of our ram, like testing a pear for ripeness.

Perhaps buying sheep is more like buying groceries than I had thought. Unquestionably though, the atmosphere is different: worse lit, different background noises, and, even at the research station, definitely more pungent.

Manure

Manure was not one of the things I considered when we were deciding to buy sheep. It had always been a nice, rich-smelling substance that came in a plastic bag and was dug into gardens. Until we got into the business of producing it. Then manure was no longer an asset, it was a problem.

I really didn't realize the extent of the problem until I brought my Campfire kids out to see the baby lambs that first spring.

"Gross!" they said.

I hadn't thought of manure as gross. I'd changed diapers for almost six years and must have grown through the "gross" stage in the first month. But nine-year-olds who had never changed a diaper in their lives and who hadn't been walking through the barnyard all winter had a different reaction.

"Gross."

"Yuck!"

"Poop."

The spring sun had turned the barnyard to mud, and rivulets of brown water made their way across the hard-packed drive and down the hill to add to the mess. Sheep hooves ground feces and mud together into a yellow-brown muck.

I bundled ten pairs of feet into plastic bags and sealed them with rubber bands. "Stay on the driveway," I instructed as we entered the barnyard.

"Gross."

"Yuck."

"Poop."

"Really," I explained, "feces is just grass and corn that's been processed by the sheep." They looked at me with blank faces.

"Poop is just what's left over after your body takes everything it needs out of the food you eat," I translated.

"Gross."

"Yuck."

"Not me!"

"Yes, even you." I never imagined in graduate school that I'd use my masters in biochemistry to explain poop to a group of disbelieving nine-year-olds.

I'm glad I only have to deal with sheep manure and not cow manure. Sheep generally produce little brown marbles of feces. Cows produce huge sloppy piles. When the sheep start producing sloppy piles, there's trouble afoot—and under foot. This became painfully clear after the arrival of six new ewe lambs in the second summer of my shepherdessing career.

Spot, one of the new lambs, started behaving strangely. She was shy and hung out in the back corner of the pasture; most unusual, she didn't come up for corn. And then one morning she was dead.

Stunned, I wrapped her body in a blanket and took her into the veterinary clinic. Dr. Hexum, grandfatherly and kind, did the autopsy for me.

"She had *Haemonchus contortus*," he said. "Worms."

I'd never heard of *"Humongous contorted."* I bought enough medicine to worm the rest of my sheep, and they stopped having the diarrhea I hadn't even noticed.

Diarrhea can be a symptom of a lethal worm problem in sheep, and my ignorance had killed a lamb. My self-incriminations were boundless. I was probably better educated than 95 percent of the population in town, and I couldn't do a simple job like farming. Lots of the farmers I'd met hadn't even finished high school, and they did a better job than I did. I vowed I'd never lose another lamb through lack of knowledge. I read more sheep books.

THE NEXT SPRING, lack of manure became a problem. I was so worried about two newborn lambs who were rejected by their mother that I barely noticed their quiet brother, who never bugged me and had a round little belly. Finally, at my 4 A.M. trip to the barn, I realized that I hadn't seen him nursing for the last twenty-four hours, since right after he was born. He was too quiet and reserved. He stood all hunched up, back arched, head down, as if he were starving.

I sat down with my pile of books and began looking for a problem to fit his symptoms. Sure enough, I found one: a meconium plug that hadn't been expelled, resulting in a buildup of gas in his belly. Meconium is the first tarry black feces an animal produces after it is born. If the meconium gets stuck in the intestines, the animal doesn't feel well and stops eating. A newborn lamb can starve to death in forty-eight hours.

I must have read that chapter a dozen times before, but meconium plugs never had any reality for me until I had to find a solution for a sick lamb.

I poured two spoonfuls of mineral oil into his mouth. Three hours later, he was starting to bounce around like a normal lamb. His belly was still big, but something was going on in there. Six hours later, he was normal-sized and nursing well, a complete cure.

EVEN WHEN IT'S produced by healthy animals, manure is a very big problem because it has to be moved out of the barn and away from the feeders. The first year, Dave and I hauled the manure-filled bedding to the garden in a wheelbarrow and dug it in. The straw and manure combination did wonderful things for the soil—much better than store-bought manure-in-a-bag.

The next year, with fourteen sheep, we had to shovel manure all winter long. The sheep never seemed to figure out that manure doesn't belong in feeders or water tanks. It belongs on the ground. I never saw the sheep dirtying their feeders or water tanks, so they must have done it in the dark of night. Every night. And every day I strained manure out of their water. We designed feeders specifically to keep manure out of their feed. To no avail. The manure piles around their feeders grew higher and higher, and the feeders seemed to sink into the ground. So we shoveled manure. By spring the lambs played king of the mountain on a five-foot-high manure pile. In September we moved the pile into the pickup and then onto the garden. That was work!

At this point, our garden had reached the saturation point, so we tried to ignore the manure buildup the next year. We raised the feeders instead of digging them out. We added fresh bedding on top of the dirty bedding. Dave began hitting his head on the barn rafters and ducking when he went through the door as the manure and straw built up on the barn floor. Then we had a warm winter and the barn reeked of ammonia. Lambs got pneumonia. I had neglected my job and the lambs were paying for it.

After lambing we borrowed a skid loader and a manure spreader from Howard, the man who used to farm our land. Howard not only loaned us equipment, he taught us how to run it and gently gave us advice. "You don't want to leave the twine from the hay bales on the ground," he'd say. "They get hung up in the spreader."

We cleaned the barn and barnyard, scraping up all the old manure and straw and unused hay and spreading it on our hayfields. It was cheaper than fertilizer and less destructive environmentally, but it was a long, tedious chore. Old baling twine kept getting tangled in the spreader, and we'd have to stop and cut it out. The house stank for two days, and people could smell our farm all the way into town.

I've heard of a shepherd who made up little cloth bags of manure with the sheep's name and picture on each bag and actually got people to buy "Persephone's Pellets" or "Fair's Feces." This was not the image I had for myself when I began raising sheep. Obviously I should have studied business instead of biochemistry. Then I wouldn't be knee-deep in manure—or I'd be making money from it. We've noticed that dogs love eating sheep manure. Perhaps we should sell it as doggie treats.

I worried when we first bought sheep that our dogs would kill them, and we carefully latched the gate every time we went through. Then one day we forgot. I looked out the kitchen window and saw the sheep ravenously eating lettuce. And the sheep-killing dogs? They were in the pasture ravenously eating sheep manure. That escape was my first hint that fences impregnable to coyotes and dogs might not be tight enough to keep sheep in. Especially hungry sheep.

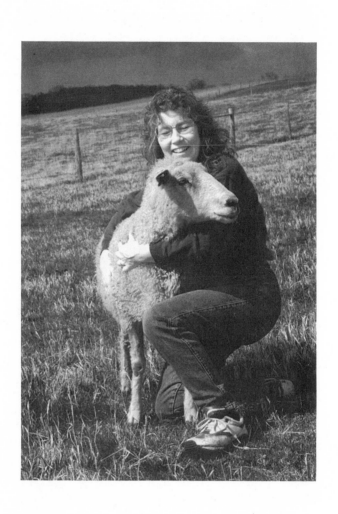

Wagging Their Tails behind Them

Dave, the sheep are gone!"

The fence was down. We saw that as we drove into the pasture, but we didn't miss the sheep until we drove over the hill. They weren't lying in their sunny hollow. They weren't grazing in the fresh alfalfa. They hadn't gone to visit the rams. They weren't in the barnyard.

"They couldn't just disappear." My voice was plaintive. "Where can they be?"

"You take the truck back along the road," Dave said. "I'll check the woods."

It was hard to drive and watch for sheep prints or sheep droppings or even sheep at the same time. I drove very slowly, stopping at every puddle to look for hoofprints. Whenever I came to a high spot on the road, I'd look across the fields for some sign of the sheep.

Two large white blobs in a neighbor's hayfield. I shaded my eyes against the sun and stared. They didn't move, not even a ripple of wool in the wind. Rocks, I decided. The puddles held only tire tracks. At two houses I put on a Bo Peep act. "Have you seen any sheep? I've lost my whole flock." I didn't think twice about exposing my ineptness. This was important. They all commiserated, but they had seen nothing.

I drove east and then west along the road that bordered our farm. Finally I drove back to the house, prey to depressing thoughts. Did our insurance cover sheep? Should I report them to the police? Where would I find replacement ewes at this time of year? No replacement ewes would have the wonderful fleeces I'd been developing.

I stopped in the pasture for a last try. "Hey ewes," I called. "Hey ewes." No hungry baaas answered me. No inquisitive noses nudged me.

Dejected, I climbed back into the truck. Thirteen ewes. Cocoa, Brownie, and Fair. Polar Bear with her babies, Puddles and Persephone, always tagging behind her. Charlie and Cinnamon, bouncy and independent. Cinder and Roses. My new ewes, Nutmeg, Mrs. McCawber, and Anonymous. All those beautiful fleeces, lost. All my friends gone.

I hadn't realized how important they were to me. Of course I felt protective of them. After all, I wanted to be the best I could at my job. But my feelings went beyond dissatisfaction at a job poorly done. I felt hurt, almost in a panic, close to how I'd felt when I lost Laurel in a mall.

Horrid visions swarmed through my mind—rustlers, dogs, coyotes, wolves!

I lectured myself. Rustlers could never catch Nutmeg. She hated people and kept her distance. We didn't have wolves in this part of Minnesota. I hadn't heard a coyote all summer long. All the neighbors' dogs were old and small. Still, the scenarios were there, circling in my brain.

They were my babies. I loved them. I loved the calm expression on Cocoa's big face, the shy look in Brownie's golden-brown eyes, little Puddles with her woolless head looking strange and unfinished.

Tears streaming down my face unchecked, I drove down the driveway. Dave came out of the barnyard. He was grinning.

"You found them!" I shouted. "Where were they?"

He laughed. "You'll never guess. They were in the front yard, eating daylilies."

LOSING THE SHEEP brought home to me how much I loved them. I loved their beautiful fleeces and their funny personalities. And I loved the idea of another lambing coming soon. Well, maybe I was also frightened by it.

The baby lambs were wonderful. The concept of delivering a lamb was not. I had learned a lot in the past year, but because the first ones had been born without my help, lambing was still an unknown, a frightening unknown, rapidly approaching.

Just as I had really learned about mothering by being a mom and had learned about worms by having a lamb die, the only way I was going to learn about lambing was to do it. But my mothering books, my parenting books, didn't say, "If you don't do this, your baby will die." The behaviors that keep human babies alive come naturally to human mothers.

The behavior I needed to keep my lambs alive didn't come naturally to me. I was a person, not a sheep. I could only read and reread my sheep books and assume that mothering behaviors came naturally to my sheep, that the instinct to mother was as strong as the instinct to breach fences to find gourmet daylilies.

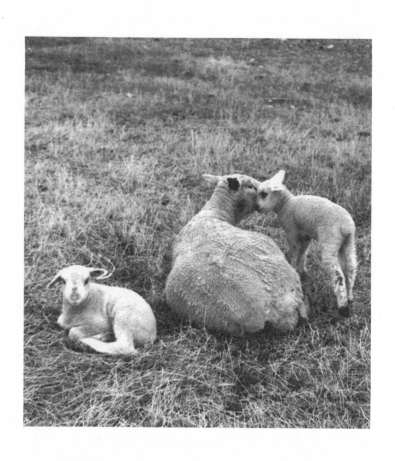

MAAA

aaa."

I stepped out of the icy wind and into the smelly warmth of the barn to Mrs. McCawber's friendly gurgle. But she wasn't talking to me. She was talking to the little white shape at her side! The lamb unfolded itself and staggered to its feet, long legs shaking as it stood for the first time. It bleated and looked wildly around for the reassuring bulk of its mother. Calmly, the ewe answered her son with another reassuring "maaa" and then returned to her work, licking another lamb! This one, a second white ram, still lay in the straw, eyes open wide, legs gathering themselves for that first effort. First the hind legs straightened. Up, then down, then up again, fighting gravity and their own weakness and inexperience. Finally his hind legs were up to stay, and he began working on the front pair. His shoulders bunched and heaved. He was up to his knees, great long forelegs still lying under him. Another heave and he was standing, legs spread wide for balance. His bleating joined the soft calls of the first lamb.

This time Mrs. McCawber didn't respond. Her head was straining forward and up, eyes shut. She grunted. From her vulva slipped a slimy bundle. Beneath the glistening transparent membrane, I could see the head of a third lamb, bony and white, with huge dark eyes. As the lamb slid to the floor, the ewe clambered to her feet and turned to sniff at the baby lying motionless in its uterine covering. The lamb twitched, its legs moved jerkily, and its head lifted slightly. Mrs. McCawber began licking her new lamb, cleaning the membrane from its mouth and nose so that it could breathe. Carefully and calmly, she licked the little body lying at her feet. Soon the membrane was gone; only a yellow yolky substance remained in the lamb's tight white curls.

When the third lamb staggered to its feet, Mrs. McCawber turned her attention to the first two babies, who were now butting purposefully at her stomach, legs, and udder, instinctively trying to satisfy their hunger. The ewe carefully nudged a hungry lamb with her nose until it was facing backward. Then she pushed on its hind end until the lamb's head ran into her udder. The lamb pushed at different parts of it until his nose brushed against a nipple. Then he butted repeatedly at the nipple until it slipped into his mouth. His body went rigid, only his mouth moving. Then a shudder started at the lamb's shoulders and rippled all the way to the tip of his long tail. As he nursed, his tail continued to wiggle with obvious contentment.

With her eldest-born quieted down, Mrs. McCawber turned to her second lamb and pushed that one into position on her other side. By the time the first lamb had finished, baby number three was sticking her head into every opening she could find between her siblings and her mother. When her brother moved away, she homed in on the udder and immediately began to nurse, tail wriggling. Within an hour, Mrs. McCawber and her three lambs were all nestled cozily in a corner, the lambs asleep, Mrs. McCawber grunting contentedly.

I hadn't realized that the ewe would know exactly what to do during lambing. I hadn't known how calm, really pastoral, the entire process was.

The sounds were pleasant, contented sounds; little grunts and low maaas from Mrs. McCawber, plaintive little baaas from the lambs. No distress from Mrs. McCawber, only obvious mothering sounds. No distress from the lambs, only statements of existence and hunger.

There was no blood. Oh, the placenta, which came out soon after lamb number three, had blood in it. But there was no bleeding, no wound. Birth really was a normal process.

Lamb number three, speckled face pressed between her mother's leg and her udder, nursed enthusiastically as her mother calmly ate the placenta. My eyes opened wide. I'd read about animals doing that, but it hadn't sunk in. Pieces of straw clung to the placenta as Mrs. McCawber ate it. I gagged, thankful that humans had lost their taste for such things.

It was the placenta that pulled me back to my role as a shepherdess instead of observer. I hadn't done any of my carefully memorized three-part lambing ritual: "clip, dip, strip."

First, the umbilical cord is clipped to one inch right after birth. Of course, I hadn't witnessed any births, so I had done it for all newborns whenever I found them. I used a knife my brother had made for me. The blade was corroding from the iodine solution used to sterilize the knife, but the handle fit my hand well. I felt good using it.

Next comes the dipping. After clipping the umbilical cord, I dip the stub into an iodine solution. Usually I hold the bottle up to the lamb's belly, stuff the cord into the mouth of the bottle, press the bottle against the belly, and then turn lamb and bottle upside down. Together. Hopefully.

I have iodine stains on my coveralls caused by wriggly lambs or lack of coordination on my part. I also managed to stain two lambs yellow from the iodine. I hoped the iodine would fade eventually; I didn't think I could sell yellow fleeces.

Finally, we strip some milk from the ewe's teats to make the initial nursing easier for the lambs. First-time mothers sometimes object to strange cold hands on their nipples. New shepherds sometimes have a hard time with the process, too.

Mrs. McCawber obviously didn't need her teats stripped. She had no problem with my picking up her babies; one under my left arm, one under my right, and the third clutched to my chest. She didn't object when I carried her lambs across the barn to the jug. She followed the baaas of her babies, sniffing and maaaing in return.

I unloaded the lambs in the jug, a four-by-four-foot space that we separated from the rest of the barn with plywood panels. The jug to the east of Mrs. McCawber held Cocoa and her iodine-stained day-old twins. To the west, Fair nursed her little black twin rams. Each ewe and her lambs were jugged for at least forty-eight hours, giving them a chance to bond with no interference.

No interference except from the shepherd, that is. I tied the front plywood panel shut, gathered my knife, iodine bottle, and towels and climbed into the jug. Kneeling in a corner, I uncapped the iodine bottle and carefully set it aside. Then I picked up a lamb, set it between my legs on its back and cut off the trailing cord. Usually I cut off two to three inches of tissue. Some ewes trimmed the cord themselves, so that all I had to do was dip it in iodine.

The iodine was important. It dried up the tissue and

kept infections from getting started in the stub. Barn floors aren't particularly clean, and newborn lambs spend most of their time lying on their bellies. I wasn't about to ignore a simple precaution.

I wasn't about to ignore any of the precautions listed in my books. The other major suggestion was to rub the lamb dry with an old bath towel. In really cold weather (and what Minnesota March is not really cold?) a wet lamb loses body heat rapidly. I've even read of lambs whose ears froze solid. Last year I kept my hair dryer in the lambing shed to dry off wet ears. But experience taught that a towel worked just as well, could be used more than two feet from the electrical outlet, and didn't scare the sheep with the noise it made.

Mrs. McCawber's lambs were all dry. They had each nursed for a second time and were curling up together for a nap. I turned on the heat lamp over their jug. It would keep them warm until morning. After that they'd keep themselves warm with no problems.

I climbed over the panel at the front of the jug, put iodine, knife, and towels away in the hanging cabinet and counted the ewes. There should be thirteen. If I didn't count thirteen, I'd have to go out and look for a ewe lambing by herself in some strange place, such as the top of a manure pile or under a feeder.

Tonight, all thirteen ewes were in the barn. Three in jugs with lambs, and the rest lying contentedly in the straw, chewing their cud or sleeping.

One last look at the new lambs, and I headed back to the house, content and exhilarated at the same time. The sky was lightening in the east. Dawn was still several hours away, but night was waning.

"What did you find?" Dave muttered as I slid my cold body into bed next to his warm one.

"Mrs. McCawber had triplets," I said. "And Dave, I saw the last one being born. It was a little girl. I'm going to keep her. I named her Ramona. It was wonderful."

"Great," he murmured.

"And I didn't remember to do anything. Mrs. McCawber took care of them all by herself." I hugged him to me, easing my icy feet between his. "I just stood there entranced, watching her mother."

"Mmmmm," Dave said. "Mmmmm."

He was asleep. Mrs. McCawber and her lambs were asleep. I smiled to myself and relaxed into sleep. "Mmmmm."

Fair Kept Eating

Sleep is a luxury during lambing. Every second of it is treasured. We sleep day and night. We check the sheep every three hours, do what needs to be done, go back to the house, lie down and fall asleep, to waken in three hours and do it all over again.

Laurel does the 7 A.M. check so I can make breakfast. She gets up at 6:30 and dresses for school. Then she puts on her snow suit and barn boots and goes out to the barn. If she finds anything unusual in the barn, she comes to get me.

Amber does the evening check while I work on dinner. Amber's old enough to pick up each lamb and watch to see if it stretches. A warm, full, comfortable lamb stretches when you pick it up. A hungry, sick lamb doesn't. If Amber finds a lamb that doesn't stretch, she comes to get me.

If Dave's home, he and I share the rest of the checks. Dave works fifteen-hour night shifts at the hospital and so functions better at night than I do. But the sheep are my responsibility, so I try to take the majority of the shifts. But after a few nights of interrupted sleep, it's really easy to turn over and slide back into sleep if Dave offers to check the sheep. Dave works for a week and then is off for ten days. During his week-long stretches at the hospital, I do all the checks and all the feeding and all the veterinary work and all the family chores. I can't imagine always doing this all by myself.

WHOEVER IS CHECKING the sheep first looks for new lambs and then for ewes in labor. Next we check for lambs who are standing all hunched up and ewes who are acting strangely or whose udders look peculiar.

Peculiar-looking udders used to mean I hadn't looked at enough udders. They all looked peculiar. But now I can recognize mastitis, a bacterial infection that, in one form, may cause a ewe to lose the milk-producing ability in half or all of her udder; and when caused by another bacterium, mastitis often results in death. It took me a long time to learn. I snuck up on a lot of ewes to touch their udders before I could differentiate between full udders and empty udders; clean udders and dirty udders; soft udders and udders swollen hard and colored dark with mastitis.

And now from a distance, Fair's udder suddenly looked unusual. One half seemed very large and dark. Fair is a friendly and hungry ewe. She's always ready to eat, which is why she weighs more than two hundred pounds. I walked into the pasture with a bucket of grain. "Hey ewes," I called, to let her know I was there. Fair's big black head rose. I rattled the grain bucket. Fair started into a lumbering run, her ears flapping out to the side. If she didn't weigh so much, she could fly with those ears.

I dumped the corn onto the ground. Fair gobbled as fast as she could, completely unconcerned about what I was doing. I was trying to take her down. I knelt beside her, reached under her body with both hands and grabbed the legs on the far side. Fair kept eating. I pushed my shoulder against Fair's shoulder and pulled on her far legs. Fair kept eating, but nothing else happened. I needed more leverage. Still holding Fair's legs, I climbed from my knees to a squat. This time when I pulled on her legs and pushed on her shoulder, she crashed to the ground. Hurriedly, I lay down on her body to keep her from getting up again. Fair stretched her neck toward the corn and kept eating.

I lay facing Fair's head. Everything I needed to do was at the other end, so I carefully and slowly swung my body around until I was facing her rear end. I felt her udder. Half of it was hot and hard. Definitely mastitis. Twelve cc of penicillin intramuscularly first. I pulled the syringe out of my shirt pocket and slid my body forward until I could brace my arms on her pelvis. I stabbed the needle into the big muscle of her thigh. Then I slowly injected the penicillin. Penicillin stings as it goes in, and I didn't know how Fair would react. My muscles were tensed, ready to counteract any move she made. Fair kept eating.

I pulled the needle out and laid the syringe on the ground beside us. Now I needed to milk Fair to empty all the parts of her udder where the bacteria might be growing. I slid closer to her tail and reached around her hind legs. Fortunately, the hard half of Fair's udder was facing up. I began massaging it, first the top, then the middle, then the bottom. Fair kept eating. I couldn't reach the top of the udder as well as I'd like, so I sat up and slid closer, my legs going around her body. "I don't know how to milk an animal," I grumbled to myself. "Why don't these things happen when Dave's home?"

Of course Dave was better at this sort of stuff, he'd had years of practice. He'd spent summers on his grandparents' dairy farm, feeding calves and milking cows. My closest encounter with farm life was a white rat in a plastic cage on the shores of Bald Eagle Lake—not sufficient training for being a milkmaid. But Fair's mastitis couldn't wait for Dave to get back; I had to milk her.

Slowly and carefully, I massaged down her udder, starting at the top again and working toward the bottom. I pulled my fingers down her teat, milk squirting out.

The udder was noticeably softer after my third pass down the udder. Perhaps I could do this myself.

Suddenly I felt Fair's muscles tense. I grabbed her back and her hind leg and thought heavy thoughts, but to no avail. Her muscles heaved, and she struggled to her feet. I was still on her back, feet dangling six inches off the ground on either side. My hands dug into her wool, fingers clenched. Just as I shifted my body to slide off, Fair lumbered forward and then broke into a run. We passed the empty bucket at a gallop.

My fingers were saying, "Hold on, hold on!" My feet were saying, "Get off, get off!" And my mind was gibbering. I pressed my head against Fair's back and watched the fence stream by. At this rate she'd soon be in the woods, and I'd be scraped off by a tree. That thought did it. My fingers relaxed, and I threw my body to the left. Fair ran right out from under me. I hit the ground with my knees and elbows, sliding to a stop. I lay on the hard ground, tears of pain and frustration starting in my eyes. Suddenly, I heard a whuffle. I opened my eyes. Fair's big ears blocked out the sun as she began munching the grass in front of my face. Painfully I got to my feet. Holding my throbbing right elbow with my scraped and bleeding left hand, I limped homeward. Some days, the rat in the cage seemed like a much better idea. After a few feet, I glanced back over my shoulder. Fair's udder looked better.

Fair kept eating.

Market Day, My Way

Eating occupies the lambs, too, all summer long. They eat grass and nurse. From the time they first find their mothers' nipples until they are weaned, they nurse. When the mood hits them, they unerringly pick their mothers out of the flock, day or night. Even after they are getting most of their nutrients from grass and spend most of the day racing across the pasture with the other lambs, they still seek out their mothers for frequent snacks. Two or three lambs often try to nurse at once, shouldering each other out of the way and butting enthusiastically at their mother's udder.

When the ewes finally tire of nursing, they wean their lambs. I can tell when it's almost time. Two almost full grown lambs converge on their mother's udder. They butt it several times, lifting their mother off the ground, and then they nurse hungrily. Mom escapes as rapidly as possible. One day soon, she won't stop when the lambs converge on her; she'll keep moving until they give up.

The lambs eat and gain weight. By October or November, they are big enough for market.

Market day, the way we sell our lambs, occurs at least once a week all through October and November. It would be less work if we took them to the teleauction or

the stockyards, and I'd only have to go through the griev-
ing process once. But it is better that we do it this way.
At least I still remember that they are animals.

When someone orders a lamb for their freezer, I
make an appointment with the butcher. Early Wednesday
morning, Dave and I load the lamb into the back of the
pickup. The drive into town is short, but by the time we
park at the back of the butcher shop, the lamb is shivering. I don't know if the truck ride scares them or if the
smell at the butcher's awakens a racial memory. I climb
into the pickup and grab the lamb, sinking my fingers into
his fleece. I hug his little body to mine and kiss him and
thank him. The Indians did that—the thanking, that is—
with the animals they killed. It seems the least I can do.

I am having troubles with my conscience. Do I really
want to raise animals for slaughter? Perhaps I should
turn vegetarian and sell my rams, only keeping the ewes
for their fleeces and not breeding them.

But I like to eat meat. And furthermore, this is a job,
not a hobby, and I need to earn enough money to pay for
the upkeep of the ewes. As it is, the farm doesn't always
make money. If I have to buy hay because the equipment
kept breaking down during haying, we don't make money.
If I have to buy a lot of lamb milk replacer to feed bottle
lambs, we don't make money. If I have the vets out for
too many sick ewes, we lose money. If I hire extra help
for fencing or haying, we lose money.

If no minor catastrophes happen, we make money. A
little bit of money. Not enough to put the kids through
college or to retire on. Not enough to live on for a year.
But enough to satisfy the IRS that I actually run a working farm. As I learn more, haying will get better, I'll need
the vets less, and we'll have fewer bottle lambs. As the
kids get older, I won't have to hire outside help. I sure

hope they continue to enjoy farming. Right now they really do. They love the lambs and the excitement of shearing and lambing. They enjoy the notoriety that having a shepherdess for a mother brings.

I take wool into my Sunday school class and talk about how they spun when Jesus was a boy. I show them the drop spindle and talk about the kind of sheep they had back then. We talk about how long it must have taken to spin enough yarn to make fabric for one piece of clothing.

I take baby lambs into Amber's and Laurel's school classes. We play with the lamb and talk about it as it runs around the room.

"Why do his feet make that noise on the floor?"

"Because hooves are hard."

"What happened to his tail?"

"I cut it off so he would be more healthy."

"What does he eat?"

"Mostly milk."

"Then why is his poop brown?" I ignore this question.

"Does wool come from lambs?"

"Yes, let me show you." And then I get out the spinning wheel and show them how to spin wool into yarn. They all loved trying to spin themselves. "Teaching a dying craft," the school calls it. Farming, I call it.

And this craft is the reason I find myself with my crisis of conscience. Perhaps my only consolation is that I give these lambs a good life. They are healthy. They stay with their mothers for a long time. They appear to be happy—though how one judges happiness in a sheep, I don't quite know.

If they are killed mercifully, after only a short time in the slaughterhouse pens, perhaps that is all I can ask.

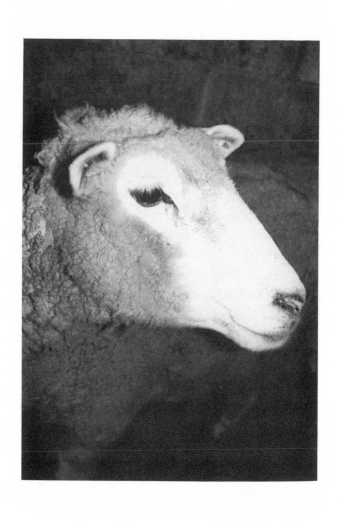

Have You Any Wool?

Shearing: constant motion from 8 A.M. until 3 P.M. tomorrow. Constant talking, constant working, a wonderful day. But everything begins today.

Incredible morning. The sun will rise soon. The sky is bands of rose and peach from the horizon on up. The colors stretch in every direction.

The temperature must be around freezing. I feel invigorated but not cold. The air is so clear! The sheep are a noisy concert of maaas and baaas. They gather around the gate waiting for me to fetch their grain.

Not yet. Just now I'm enjoying the sunrise and the silence. But how can I call it silence with the sheep baaing loudly to my left, the dogs barking joyously to my right, and two different birds calling up above me? But with all those sounds, the morning still has silence. No cars, trucks, or snowmobiles. No people. Just me and the outdoors.

Feeding today will be different. I have to shut the ewes into the barn so their fleeces will be dry. The only easy way to get them all in there is to feed them their grain in the barn. When they're hungry, they'll follow that bucket almost anywhere.

We also have to set the barn up for shearing. We'll

43

blockade the area with the scale using three-foot-high hog panels. Then we'll roll out the carpet—literally—for the shearer, make sure the broom, magic marker, forty cardboard boxes, several garbage cans, and an old bed sheet are in position. We'll hang the heat lamps so that Sonny, the shearer, can see.

Edith is bringing lasagne. I've made cookies. Coffee will go in the thermos in the morning. Milk, pop, and water are in the fridge. I want tomorrow to be smooth so that we all enjoy ourselves.

SONNY, A HUSKY sixty-five-year-old, arrives at 8 A.M. Before I am ready, always before I'm ready. He pulls into the barnyard and begins unloading his equipment: motor, shearing arm, shearing heads, toolbox, and coffee thermos.

He nails his motor to the wall above the carpet, positioning it at the top of his reach. The jointed shearing arm reaches to the floor like a giant one-legged spider.

Dave and I do last-minute chores. I find the marker for labeling boxes. Dave finds the hoof shears and fills syringes with medications.

We both keep an eye on Sonny. We want him to be happy. That means having a ewe ready for him when he's ready for her. Sonny adjusts the clippers, spits tobacco, oils the joints in the shearing arm, spits tobacco, and oils the clippers. Last year it was so cold that we had to hang a heat lamp over the shearing arm to warm the oil so that it would run. This year, at twenty degrees, we'll be quite comfortable, and the clippers will work well.

Dave guides Ramona, the first ewe, between the hog panels and onto the carpet. Sonny kneels while shearing part of each sheep, and the carpet helps his knees stay warm. It is also supposed to keep the fleeces cleaner. But I wonder—it is so dirty.

Finally, in our third year of shearing, we have a proper floor for shearing—manure! The first year, I proudly bedded our little shed with fresh straw, twenty-four hours before shearing.

"What did you do that for?" grumbled Sonny. "All that straw will mess up the fleeces." He was right. I must have picked a bale of straw out of the fleeces that first year.

The next February, I remembered that something about shearing and straw was important, but I couldn't remember what. Cleaning four fleeces obviously hadn't made much of an impression on me. I again bedded our slightly larger, jury-rigged lambing shed with straw just before we locked the sheep in.

Sonny said, "What did you do that for?" And then I remembered that the important idea was to keep the straw out of the fleeces, not to make the floor soft and warm for Sonny's knees. That winter I was grateful that Sonny brought a grungy green carpet.

The next summer, we built a proper barn. I bedded it as soon as it was done and let the straw age. By February, the floor was covered with manure. I knew Sonny would be pleased. "Nice barn," he said when he walked in. "No straw."

Sonny shears each sheep in exactly the same way. He sets Ramona on her rump more easily than Dave and I ever manage to. Then he leans her back against his legs and begins cutting the wool on her forehead. Then around her ears, the top of her head, and her cheeks. Next he shears down the sides of her head to the base of her throat and continues the path down the front of her body.

He starts at the shoulder next, clipping the left front leg and side, and then the right. As he works, the fleece peels back from Ramona's body like a heavy blanket, exposing light pink skin beneath a fine short coat of white.

Sonny works down her belly until both hind legs are shorn. He's careful around her nipples. When the nipples appear, pink and fat from beneath the wool, he grins. "This one's pregnant."

I cheer. Shearing is my first real clue as to who is pregnant and who is not. This is the real beginning of lambing. The festivities and pleasant excitement of shearing always get lambing off to a good start.

Next, Sonny lays Ramona on her side, straddles her head, and begins shearing the side to the backbone. Like many ewes, she gets restive at this point and starts pedaling her legs, but she relaxes when I hold her head off the ground. This job gives a good indication about what sheep people are like. Sonny is kneeling on the ground with a ewe's head between his legs. The helper's job is to kneel behind him and hold the sheep's head slightly off the ground. How many men want to have a sheep's head pressed against their butt by a woman they see once a year? And how many women would be willing to do the pressing?

Amazingly, raising Ramona's head just a few inches quiets her immediately. The sheep are incredibly docile during shearing. They rest quietly against Sonny's legs while he runs a whirring, pulling, cutting machine around their eyes and ears, armpits and nipples. Any human would run screaming from the room in that situation. Maybe sheep don't have enough imagination.

Yearlings—those lambs who are almost a year old and are being sheared for the first time—sometimes panic. Then the helper pulls gently but firmly out on one of their hind legs, and they quiet down. If sheep weren't calm during shearing, wool would never have become the important fiber that it is today. I can't imagine shearing a buffalo or a tiger.

When the left side is done, Sonny grabs Ramona's legs and rolls her over onto her right side. Half a minute later, he runs the clipper down her backbone and off the tail—the last cut.

Sonny rises to his feet, moves back off the sheep and gives her a push toward her feet. The ewe is off, leaving Sonny crouched over a huge pile of wool—like a sheep turned inside out; dirty gray on the inside, lustrous creamy white on the outside.

The wool is gorgeous stuff—soft, shiny, lightly crimped fibers that smell like sheep, a good smell, and still hold some of the warmth of Ramona's body. I gather it in my arms and stuff it into a box labeled Polar Bear. In my enthusiasm over the wool, I don't even realize my mistake until we shear Polar Bear.

By now, Wendy, Allen, Edith, and Gavin have come. Out of the sheep business themselves, Wendy and Allen still enjoy shearing. Wendy takes over as Sonny's helper. They have an ongoing battle of wits, resumed with no hesitation every February. "Looks like you need shearing," Sonny grunts as he waves the clippers at Wendy's curly blonde hair.

"You'll have to catch me first." Wendy grins as she catches a flailing hoof and holds it out taut. "I can catch a little girl like you," Sonny scoffs as he begins shearing Cocoa's forehead.

"No, you can't," Wendy answers. "You're too old to catch me."

Wendy and Sonny tease each other for the next six hours, making shearing enjoyable for both of them.

Allen catches Persephone and holds her for Sonny.

Dave recatches Ramona and sets her on her rump. We haven't learned Sonny's technique yet, so Dave always has problems with this maneuver. He's always eventually successful, but by afternoon, the last half dozen sheep all seem incredibly long-legged, heavy, and stubborn.

Once settled against Dave's legs, Ramona is patient while Gavin trims her hooves and I give her shots. Laurel collects each fleece and puts it into a properly labeled box. Amber and Edith skirt the dirty wool from the fleeces.

Sheep are messy animals. They get hay in their fleeces by sticking their heads under the hay piles when they eat. They get hay in their neighbors' fleeces by eating over their neighbors' backs and dribbling hay into their neighbors' wool. Hand spinners don't enjoy spinning dirty wool and won't pay well for it. So every year we skirt the fleeces—that is, we pull the dirty areas of wool from them.

Edith and Amber spread each fleece out on a wire mesh table. They shake the fleece to allow hay and straw bits to fall out. Then they remove the wool around the neck and along the back that still has hay in it. They pull off the locks from the back end of the sheep that are caked in manure. They tease out the wool locks that have somehow gotten tangled with thistles or burrs in spite of my attempts to keep the pastures weed-free. When Edith and Amber are done, the fleeces are ready to be weighed and sold.

When half of the sheep are sheared, we break for lunch. Amber and Laurel have the table set, sandwich fixings sliced, and cookies arranged on a plate. We pull the lasagne from the oven and sit around the table eating hungrily. We talk about the fleeces, the sheep, and anything else in the world that seems important. Sonny takes pride in his conservative approach to life and harasses the liberal majority. Wendy baits him back. They work as a team, pulling topics out of the air for congenial argument. After we've criticized each other's views completely, we pull on our jackets and boots and head out to the barn to finish shearing the flock.

Eight P.M. finds me exhausted and ecstatic. We've sheared, medicated, and pedicured forty sheep. Their fleeces are all skirted, weighed, and ready to sell. The sheep are fed and shut in the barn for warmth overnight.

A sinkful of dirty dishes waits for me. But that's in the house. I'm in the barn, where the lights throw some ewes into stark relief and some into shadow. I listen to the ewes, look at their pregnant bellies, check for fat udders. The world is just me and the sheep. Only the lambs are missing, and they'll come soon.

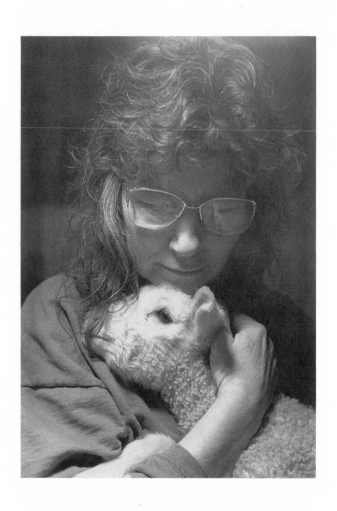

Roses' Baby

The noise intruded. Why was Benny Goodman playing in our bedroom at this time of night? I looked at the clock—3:24. Consciousness drifted away, and then the music intruded again, this time Dave Brubeck's "Take Five." The clock said 3:44. Why was jazz playing in our bedroom at 3:44 in the morning? Slowly, my brain awoke. The alarm had been set for three o'clock. I was more than forty minutes late. I had to go out to the barn.

Pushing the covers back, I forced myself to sit up. Shivering with cold and limp as a rag doll, I collapsed back on the bed and drifted back toward sleep. When the radio clicked off at four, I clambered to my feet and began pulling on clothes—socks, sweatpants, hooded sweatshirt. I staggered through the dark, quiet house, avoiding chairs and piles of toys by instinct. Down the stairs, right turn into the mudroom, find the barn coveralls by feel and lay them on the floor. I slipped my feet into the legs and shrugged the top up over my shoulders. Arms into the armholes. Like dressing a child, I talked myself through the process. Up with the zipper, feet into boots, mittens from the drawer into my pocket, flashlight into the other pocket.

The wind grabbed at me as I stepped outside, stealing the last of my warm sleepiness. The stars were icy sparks of light in the sky. The full moon cast shadows of trees across the yard. Warm light beckoned me from the barn. I was awake. I felt good.

Last night three newborns greeted me when I made my 3 A.M. trip to the barn. What would I find tonight?

Ewes rushed out of the barn as I entered, one trailing the bloody remnant of a placenta behind her. A new lamb was lying by himself in a depression in the straw. His little wet body was shivering. I opened the gate to a lamb pen and turned on a heat lamp.

Roses, the lamb's mother, returned to the barn and sniffed at her baby. She was very skittish. When I approached her to move the lamb, she dashed out of the barn again. I laid the lamb in his pen under the heat lamp and set off after the ewe. I drove her into the barn and toward the pen, but she avoided it time after time. The lamb was unnaturally quiet, and his mother was not yet drawn to him.

Finally I returned the lamb to the spot where he was born. I squatted beside him in the straw, waiting for Roses to return. I watched the lamb. The big eyes in his little face didn't open. He wasn't struggling to get to his feet. And he seemed so cold. Deep inside me, worry started to grow.

Roses rushed back to the spot where she lambed. She sniffed the little black bundle at her feet, watching me warily. I reached for the lamb again. "It's okay," I told her. "I'm trying to help you." Voice slow and soft, I continued talking as I moved backward toward the pen, crouching low with the lamb held out for Roses to see and smell. "See, here's your baby. Come on, come with your baby." Roses was moving. I glanced over my shoulder. Another four feet, and we'd be in the pen. "It's okay, Roses. It's all right. Come and get your baby."

Eventually I bumped into the wall and laid the lamb in the far corner of the pen. As I climbed over the partition into an adjoining pen, Roses approached her lamb. She sniffed it, licked it. The lamb raised its head blindly and then let it flop back onto the straw bedding. Roses looked up as if puzzled. Her instincts didn't tell her what to do for a lamb that didn't fight for life.

I swung the gate to the pen shut and reviewed what I had to do for the lamb. "Clip, dip, strip." That litany had gotten me through two years of lambing: clip the umbilical cord, dip it in iodine, strip the ewe's teats so the milk flowed. But none of these would help a lamb that wasn't normal. They wouldn't help him open his eyes or lift his head or stand up.

The worry inside of me swelled into a big cloud of fear. I could feel the panic in my chest pushing against my lungs. It was hard to breathe. My heart was pounding. My mouth was dry. I didn't know what to do for this lamb. My experience didn't help me. My books couldn't help me.

Grabbing a towel, I clambered back into the pen. I frightened Roses, but she'd just have to put up with it. At least I could make the lamb warm and dry. I crouched under the heat lamp with the tiny shivering body cradled in my hands and tried to rub his wool dry. Tried to rub some life into him. Even lying in my hands, he didn't feel right. His neck was stiff, not flexible like all the other lambs I'd held. His eyes didn't open, and he didn't cry for his mother.

When his shivering stopped, I laid him in the straw in the circle of light and warmth thrown by the heat lamp. My chest was still tight, tears were very near. This lamb was not healthy, and I didn't know what to do. I took one last look to make sure he was breathing and headed for the house and for help.

53

ARMED WITH MY reference books and a bottle of colostrum, Dave and I walked slowly back to the barn. My
heart was pounding, emotions under tight control. I must
not panic. I couldn't help this lamb if I panicked.

Dave picked up the little black body. The lamb was
still breathing, but he was shivering again. Dave held it
close under the heat lamp as I filled a stomach feeder
with colostrum. The stomach feeder, a big syringe with
a long flexible plastic tube instead of a needle, was used
to give a lamb milk when it didn't have the strength to
nurse. I reread the section on stomach feeding in my
book, then I ran my fingers along the lamb's mouth, trying to open it. His jaw was as stiff as his neck. Finally I
forced an opening big enough for the quarter-inch plastic tube and slipped the tube in.

"Remember to keep the tube toward the back of his
throat."

Dave's voice startled me. I stopped. The fear and
panic almost overwhelmed me. I didn't want the lamb to
die. But I could kill it myself if I squirted milk into his
lungs instead of his stomach.

"I'm so afraid."

"Just keep the tube toward the back. You're doing
fine."

Holding the lamb's head, I fed more of the tube into
his mouth. His breathing didn't change, he didn't cough
or gag. When almost ten inches of the tube were inside
the lamb, I slowly pushed the plunger on the syringe,
filling the lamb's belly with warm, life-giving colostrum.
I pulled the tube out and sat back on my heels.

The lamb lay quietly, his little chest rising and falling
as he breathed, head still, eyes closed. I looked at Dave.
The light fell on his head as he knelt, looking down at the
lamb in his hands. Momentarily, I forgot the lamb. This

wasn't Dave's job. He had been working nights for a week. This was his time to sleep well. But he had gotten up in the middle of the night to help me with Roses' baby. A warm rush of love overwhelmed me. Then Dave lifted his head and his face moved out of the shadow. I could see his expression.

"He's dying, isn't he?" My voice broke.

"I'm afraid so. His breathing is more uneven."

"The colostrum didn't help." I pressed my forehead against my hands. I didn't want him to die, and I couldn't do anything about it.

Dave put the lamb down. "I think we might as well go into the house," he said.

"If we go in, he won't be alive in the morning."

"Joanie, he won't be alive in the morning if we stay out here, either. His breathing is getting worse all the time." Dave looked at me across the body of the little black lamb. "Do you want to watch him die?"

The tears were streaming down my face. I shook my head. I touched his little black head and got tiredly to my feet. Turning to the ewe, I thought of how I would have felt if my babies had died. I thought of how confused she must be. "I'm sorry, Roses," I said. "I'm so sorry."

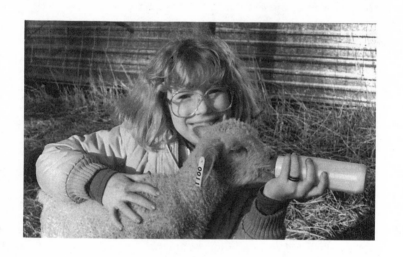

Crazy 8

The death of Roses' baby haunted me. I had been incompetent. I read and reread the lambing books looking for answers.

When Anonymous's second lamb, number 8, didn't show any interest in nursing and cried piteously and continuously, I knew I couldn't lose another lamb. I tucked him, a limp, wet bundle, inside my jacket and carried him into the house. Amber and Laurel spread towels in front of the woodstove. We laid him on the towels, and the girls offered him a bottle of colostrum.

Colostrum is the first milk that an animal produces after birthing and is full of the antibodies necessary to babies. Every year I found a dairy farmer with excess colostrum and begged some to have on hand. If number 8 had been nursing on his mother, he would have gotten his colostrum from her.

At first number 8 wouldn't nurse on the bottle, either. But after Laurel poked the nipple into his mouth, he stopped crying and sucked hungrily.

It was great fun having a lamb in the house. Amber and Laurel dried him and cuddled him until he struggled out of their arms and stood uncertainly on his feet. He rapidly progressed to bouncing around the living room and kitchen. His little white hooves clattered on the tile. The girls named him Crazy 8, just to have something to call him in the house.

When Crazy 8 stopped to urinate, I decided it was time for him to go back to his mother. He was definitely a success story.

He had only been in the house two hours, but in that time he had changed from a weak, almost lifeless newborn to a fuzzy white lamb that staggered around curiously, alert and full of life.

The change was too much for Anonymous. She sniffed him carefully from head to tail. She sniffed her other lamb and then resniffed Crazy 8. Then she butted Crazy with her head, hard.

He slammed against the wall of the pen. Crazy got to his feet and headed for his mother's udder. As he passed her nose, she sniffed his tail and then tossed him across the pen again.

I cuffed Anonymous on the head and shouted at her. Crazy 8 climbed to his feet and headed for her udder. Again she pushed him out of the way and turned her back on him.

Crazy whimpered, his sister whimpered, and Anonymous muttered her mothering sounds while sniffing Crazy's sister. Crazy scampered under his mother's body and butted her udder with his nose, searching for a nipple. Without pausing in her sniffing, Anonymous moved sideways, leaving Crazy in the open. He approached his mother's udder again. She sidestepped. Then, whipping her head around, she shoved Crazy 8 aside.

"Stop it!" I shouted. "He's your baby, just like the other one!" I grabbed her head and held on tight. Crazy 8 approached her udder again, more carefully this time. When his mother didn't move, he grabbed a teat in his mouth and sucked.

When Crazy 8 stopped nursing, I released Anonymous's head. She ignored him. I began my barn rounds, checking to see that each ewe had water and hay. Then I looked around the barnyard for new lambs. As I passed the barn door, I heard the thunk of Crazy 8 hitting the jug wall again.

I dashed across the barn and reached the jug just in time to see Anonymous toss Crazy 8 again. "Stop it!" I shouted. I hit Anonymous on the head. The hardness of the hit brought tears to my eyes, but Anonymous didn't even notice that I had hit her.

I grabbed her head and held it to my chest, giving Crazy another chance to nurse.

For the next week, we kept Anonymous and her babies jugged, hoping that Crazy 8 would eventually smell so much like his sister that his mother wouldn't be able to tell them apart. But every time we went to the barn, we could hear the thunks as Anonymous tossed him against the wall. The only way Crazy 8 could nurse was when we held her head. We tried tying Anonymous's head in the corner, but then she kicked him away from her. She couldn't smell him, but she knew when he approached her udder.

We supplemented his diet with lamb milk replacer in a bottle three times a day. "Why isn't Anonymous taking care of him?" Laurel asked.

"I'm not sure if it's because she's a good mother or a bad mother," I said.

"What?"

59

"Well, my first guess is that she's a bad mother because she's only taking care of one baby. But she might be such a good mother that she won't waste any of her milk on a lamb that doesn't smell like her own and came after her first baby. I don't know," I said. "I can't think like a sheep."

"I'm glad you don't act like a sheep," Laurel said.

"Why?"

"Because I was your second baby!"

I laughed and gave her a hug. Then I held Anonymous's head and Laurel pushed Crazy 8 toward her udder to nurse.

Finally we turned Anonymous and her babies into the group pen and increased Crazy 8's feedings of lamb milk replacer. The group pen is a place for ewes and their two-day-old lambs to meet other sheep. The lambs learn how to recognize their mothers and not to bother other sheep. The lambs and ewes in the group pen always make a lot of noise. The ewes soon learn to recognize their babies' sounds, and the lambs learn to run toward their mothers' baaas.

The first day Crazy 8 was in the group pen, he baaaed constantly and sucked eagerly on the bottle. But each day after that, he cried less and took less milk from the bottle. I was afraid he was starving. But he looked healthy. His belly was round, and he bounced instead of walking.

Once the lambs and their mothers moved out of the group pen, we fed the lambs on a sucker bucket. The sucker bucket was a five-gallon plastic pail with six holes drilled around the middle. Six big nipples fit into the holes on the outside, and six long plastic tubes ran to the bottom of the bucket on the inside. I filled the bucket with cold lamb milk replacer twice a day.

The bottle lambs loved the sucker bucket and climbed all over me when I brought fresh milk. All except for Crazy 8. If he hadn't looked so healthy, I would have worried.

The mystery was solved one day when I sat down in a snow bank to relax after feeding the ewes. I leaned back, eyes shut, listening to the ewes eating, pigeons cooing in the barn, and water dripping somewhere—the first sign of spring.

Suddenly, all our bottle lambs were bouncing on me, their adoptive mother, looking for bottles. All the bottle lambs except for Crazy 8. When I looked around for him, he was nursing on Fair! As I watched, he moved down the row of ewes at the hay feeder to Persephone.

Crazy 8 didn't need me for an adoptive mother, he had adopted the entire flock!

My anger at Anonymous hadn't helped Crazy 8 much, but his determination to survive had been enough.

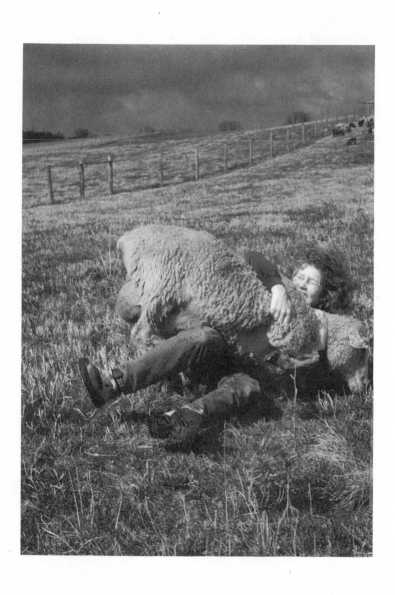

Success

Success as a shepherd can be measured in many different ways. How many ewes lambed. How many lambs lived. How well you come to know your sheep. How well you can move your sheep.

I really feel I'm a success when I manage to move the sheep by myself. Laurel and Amber were at school. Dave was at work. I had to take lambs to market that morning.

There were six lambs in the barn. All I had to do was squeeze them into the corner of the barn by the ramp and then chase them up the ramp and into the pickup.

I placed the hog panels carefully, building a funnel that ended at the ramp. The hog panels, three-foot by sixteen-foot sections of wire mesh, are slightly flexible but strong. I can carry one easily. They fit between the posts in the barn and adequately fence in the sheep.

I tied each panel once with baling twine—not really enough, as I usually use two ties per panel. But there were only six sheep, and they were only lambs.

Everything was ready. I slowly walked around behind the lambs, encouraging them into the funnel. They obediently moved to the opening of the funnel, but then they broke to the right and circled around me. I circled around them, and we started moving toward the entrance of the funnel again.

When you work sheep alone, you have to be very calm. If you get excited, they get excited and run circles around you—literally. With two or more people working, you can have a person at each spot where the sheep would typically break away, for example, at the entrance to the funnel.

Talking quietly, I started walking toward the funnel again. "It's okay. You're just going to the truck. It's all right."

Despite popular opinion to the contrary, sheep are not dumb. I used to think they were dumb back when I only had four sheep. But now that I've got thirty-five of them, I realize that on the topics of interest to sheep, they are really very intelligent and incredibly stubborn. They know when their grass supply is gone and they can spot the weakest point in the fence to destroy as they move to fresh grass. They know that they need salt and will destroy their salt feeder to tell me that the salt is all gone. They know that they should be fed before noon on winter days, and they line up noisily in front of the feeding yard to remind me of the time.

They know that four-footed creatures who bark are not sheep, and they'll try to scare them away. They know that lamb-sized four-footed creatures who meow instead of bleat are not sheep but are harmless and coexist peacefully with them. They know that two-footed creatures are generally reliable but sometimes behave strangely and are not to be trusted then. They know that pickup trucks are generally bad places to be and that open barns are generally good places.

I was trying to move the sheep out of the barn and into the pickup truck. I had to persuade the sheep that in this one case, I was to be trusted and that I knew better than they did and that they should heed my wisdom.

I was working at a disadvantage. I was lying.

It wasn't a little white lie. It was a life and death sort of lie. When I said, "It's okay. You're going to the pickup truck. It's all right," they easily perceived the contradiction and decided to go with their racial knowledge. The hell with the shepherdess.

This kind of situation teaches you how smart sheep really are. It also raises grave questions about the worth of college degrees.

I had one extra hog panel, a step stool, and a small dog. There were three places in the barn where the sheep might break away from me. The hog panel would obviously be best extending the funnel, covering the opening closest to the truck. I set Strider, our Bouvier puppy, in the middle of the second sixteen-foot opening. He wasn't really ready for this kind of work yet. He would only stay if not distracted, and the sheep were certainly distracting. But he would seem like more of a threat to the sheep than the step stool, which then divided the last sixteen-foot opening in the barn in half.

If I could keep the sheep to one side of those barriers, they would move into the funnel quite nicely. Talking softly again, I moved the sheep past the step stool and past the first post. They stopped to look at Strider. He was so cute, sitting there with his ears perked and his intelligent brown eyes watching the lambs. Then he barked, just once, and headed for the corner of the barn, with the lambs right behind him.

Unfortunately, it was the wrong corner of the barn, the one behind me. I called Strider to me, praised his courage, and told him to stay. I moved behind the sheep again and started them walking down the illusory chute.

65

They were no longer calm. They recognized the deadliness of my implacability. They didn't like the dog. They didn't like the stool much, either. They broke to the right, knocked the stool down, and gathered behind me again.

The sheep were easily winning this contest of wills. I was tired, they weren't. I was mad, they weren't. They knew what I wanted them to do, and they didn't like it. They held all the cards. Except one. I knew they could be bribed. I climbed the ladder to the hay mow, at the end of the barn, near the pickup. I threw them one bale of hay down the chute and onto the barn floor. Six lambs rushed down the funnel and clustered around the hay, six feet from the loading ramp.

I followed them with a section of hog panel, squeezing them into a six-foot square in front of the ramp. They ignored me, intent on the hay. I grabbed a handful of hay and tossed it onto the ramp. They ignored me and the hay. I grabbed the nearest lamb by the fleece and forced her up the ramp.

All the books say not to grab sheep by the fleece. It weakens the fiber, and I'm sure it hurts. But rapidly grabbing a sheep by any other part of its body is like trying to grab a running barrel, unless you are willing to throw yourself on the floor and grab feet. With my ewes, I spend a lot of time on the floor because I really don't want to damage their fleeces and I love them. But I wasn't keeping these lambs; moreover, I was extremely frustrated, and I didn't particularly want to damage myself for them. So I grabbed fleeces.

The ramp was too steep for the sheep to walk it easily. We hadn't gotten around to adding cleats, so the sheep slipped as I pushed them up the ramp. Two, three, five sheep on the ramp. But nobody was going the last

66

foot over the top and into the pickup. Everybody was turning around to face me.

Strider barked happily as lamb number six squeezed between a poorly tied hog panel and the door frame and escaped into the barnyard. No time to worry about him. I formed the bottom door of a room three feet by four feet, floor sloping up at a sixty-degree angle, and the sheep were heading down. Feet braced on the side walls, I started turning sheep. If just one would go into the truck, the rest would follow. I slowly forced my way up the ramp, pushing lambs ahead of me. Four feet is a long way to go under those conditions. Finally, the first sheep stumbled backward into the pickup. Fresh straw on the floor, light, no shepherd to harass her—a real haven. She dashed away from the ramp, and her cohorts followed her. Panting, I threw myself off the ramp and slammed the gate of the pickup shut. Five in, one to go.

I opened the funnel and the barn door. Strider and I walked into the barnyard. It was a cold, clear day. The puddles from yesterday's rain were covered with a thick layer of ice. I peeled off my jacket and gloves. My T-shirt was wet with sweat under my arms and between my breasts. How could five lambs be so much work?

Lamb number six was back in the barn calmly eating by the time my pulse returned to normal. Strider and I closed the door and easily penned the lamb with a hog panel. I couldn't use the ramp for this lamb. If I left the pickup gate open long enough to move lamb number six up the ramp, lambs one through five would come down the ramp. I was going to have to lift the lamb into the truck. That required a leg catch.

I only bruised my knees slightly as I threw myself at the lamb, grabbing her left hind leg. I shifted my grip to her underarms and stood up. This was no lamb. She was a full-grown sheep! With her back against me, my arms around her middle, she stood as tall as I did. I couldn't quite lift her feet off of the ground, so her leverage was excellent. We danced around the barn, backward. Suddenly, I backed into the water trough. I lost my balance and sat down into six inches of cold, slimy water with a sheep in my lap.

Shifting my grip again, I cradled the sheep to my chest like a very large baby. I heaved us out of the water and staggered toward the pickup. Water was running down my legs, one hundred pounds of fleece and legs flailing in my face. I tried to roll the lamb over the gate and into the back of the pickup, but I couldn't lift her high enough.

I don't very often regret being five feet two inches tall, but this was one of those times. I hitched my arms as high as possible and tried again. Still not high enough. My arm muscles were beginning to quiver.

I braced my foot on the bumper and rested the lamb on my knee. I figured I could try one more time. If I didn't make it, the lamb would ride in the cab with Strider and me. Stretching, on tiptoes, I lifted, forcing my arms as high as possible. A little longer. A little higher. Over she went!

Ninety minutes from start to finish! Shepherdess again outsmarts sheep.

Under the Haystack

utsmarting the sheep is one thing, outsmarting the weather is something else entirely. Every farmer needs to outsmart the weather: plant the field before the rains come, combine the oats before they fall off the stem, get the animals into the barn before the hail falls, bale the hay before it gets too ripe or too dry or too wet. Every farmer tries to outsmart the weather, and none of us succeed. All we can do is work with it and hope that this time at least it will all work out for the best.

Haying is different every year. Always fraught with frustration, indecision, and dependence on the weather; but otherwise different. So many factors have to come together to make a good hay crop: enough rain to make the alfalfa grow, cutting it at the correct time, no rain while the hay is drying, enough people to bale it well, and machinery that doesn't break down.

Every year we first have to work around the problem of people. Dave works seven nights in the emergency room and then is off for eleven. Ideally, we should begin baling at the beginning of his eleven-day free stretch. For that the alfalfa has to be cut at least two days before he comes home.

Cutting alfalfa is a delightful job. I have to be careful

not to crash the haybine into the large rocks embedded in the field. I have to judge carefully to cut the greatest amount of alfalfa possible without tangling the equipment in the fence at the edge of the field. And I have to make the corners neat enough to meet neighborhood standards.

If four or five days of clear weather are predicted, I cut the alfalfa just as it starts to bloom. Driving the tractor along the cut edge of the field, I see alfalfa flowers in colors from almost white with a pale tinge of purple through the lavenders to deep, deep purple. Lemon-yellow sulphur butterflies dart up out of the foliage as my creaking, groaning, clanking, roaring haybine approaches.

A rabbit darts across the stubbly field away from me. I stop the tractor and climb down. I don't want to run over a rabbit nest. I walk through the thigh-high plants but find no babies. The rabbit must have been browsing breakfast. One year, a mallard flew up as the haybine approached. We left her nest in the middle of an uncut patch of alfalfa.

The first year we cut alfalfa and put up hay, we went low-tech. Dave tilled a quarter-acre field with our tiller. Then I sowed alfalfa seed with a lawn seeder. When the alfalfa was ready, Dave cut it with a scythe we'd found at an auction. I raked the hay into windrows and turned the windrows over the next day. When the hay was dry, I drove the pickup truck through the field while Dave forked the hay into the truck. When the truck was full, Dave forked the hay out of the truck and around a ten-foot pole anchored in the ground. As Dave stacked the hay around the pole, I walked on it to pack it down.

We built two eight-foot hay stacks that way. By the time we were finished, I was clutching the pole as I walked around and around it—eight feet off the ground is not my best altitude. Then I slid down the stacks into Dave's arms.

And what beautiful hay! The stacks looked just like Little Boy Blue's. For four sheep, that was a perfectly acceptable and quite enjoyable way to bale hay. For fourteen sheep, it would be neither acceptable nor enjoyable.

The second year we had sheep, Howard, our farmer mentor, cut and baled the hay for us. Then we had to drive around the field, pulling a wagon behind the pick-up, and pick up the fifty-pound rectangular bales. Howard began baling about noon. I drove along behind the baler, stopping at each bale. Dave jumped off of the wagon, tossed the bale onto the wagon and then climbed back on. Amber dragged the bale to the back of the wagon, where Dave stacked it. Laurel played with dolls in the cab of the truck.

Dave and I were attending a party that evening, so we quit at about five o'clock. Howard kept baling. As Howard finished baling, it began to rain. We got more than two inches of rain that night, and the bales were soaked.

Wet hay molds and rots. While it's molding and rotting, it heats up. If the hay gets too hot, it can spontaneously combust, and you can lose your barn. If your sheep eat moldy hay, they can abort. Our wet bales of hay were a real disaster.

We tried to dry them by turning every bale on edge. The next day we leaned the bales against each other in piles of four. Every day we lifted the bales and slid our hands inside them, hoping to find that they were light and dry. They kept feeling heavy, wet, and hot. Finally we painfully loaded all those wet, heavy bales into the truck and unloaded them at the side of the field. We saved them "just in case" we needed them. The next summer,

Amber and Laurel and I moved those bales for the fifth and sixth time to an eroding gully along our road. At least this hay, which had absorbed so much water, could absorb some more to the benefit of our road.

The second time we baled hay that summer, we called a lot of friends to help and kept picking up the bales until we were done. It was back-breaking work. Every bale had to be lifted at least three feet to get it onto the wagon, and the top row of bales on the wagon was more than eight feet high. Dave could toss a bale up there by himself. I had to boost it onto the wagon and then push it up one layer of bales at a time. We wore out friends rapidly that summer.

The third year we bought our own baler. It was an incredible collection of dirty green pieces of metal clanking and banging together, plastered with notices saying, in essence, "Don't do anything to anything while anything is moving or might move."

I took the notices at face value and didn't touch the baler.

When the hay was ready, we called all the friends who had shown the least interest in repeating their baling experience. Only three people could fit us into their schedules. Dave drove the tractor, and six of us climbed onto the wagon being pulled behind the baler, which was being pulled behind the tractor.

When the first bale moved off the chute of the baler and onto the wagon, I grabbed it and backed toward the back of the wagon. I collided with Amber, who grabbed Laurel as she stumbled toward the edge of the wagon.

"Stop!" we shouted to Dave. We conferred and decided that six was too many people on the wagon. We dispatched the girls to the house to make something cool to drink.

Dave's brother Paul grabbed the next bale and knocked Mike off the wagon when he swung the bale around.

"Stop!" we shouted. Four people was still too many. I went to help the girls until there was a load of hay ready to unload into the barn. Mike, Gavin, and Paul were able to coexist on the wagon without knocking each other off and get the hay stacked, too.

Building a load is an exercise in three-dimensional problem solving. Our wagon holds five bales placed side by side across its width and four bales end to end, front to back. Depending on how well the bales are made and how carefully each layer is arranged, the wagon can be four, five, or even six layers high.

Our six-layer loads always seem to come at the very end of a long, hot day. "Let's quit," Dave said late one afternoon.

"There are only about twenty more bales," I argued. "Let's finish."

We managed to get all the bales onto the wagon. Halfway down the hill, on the home stretch, the load began to sway. Each swing grew a little wider. By the third cycle, the load didn't recover. In slow motion, forty or fifty bales fell off the wagon and spread themselves along the hillside.

After five years of experience on Dave's and my part, and five years of growing by the girls, we finally arrived at the best way to bale hay. The four of us do it by ourselves. That way we only have to be concerned with our schedules and the weather. Dave drives, Amber grabs bales and drags them to me, and I stack them. Laurel redistributes the hay from broken bales into windrows and helps haul bales. When the load is done, four layers high—no more!—we drop Laurel off at the house to make cold drinks and cookies. Then I throw the bales onto the bale elevator, which carries them into the barn. Amber and Dave stack them in the barn. After Laurel brings out the refreshments, she helps move bales to the elevator. If we want to work twice as fast, we can use two people on the wagon loading bales and three people at the barn unloading. Gavin offers to help every year. Of course we always accept outside help.

Friends are an important part of farming. I'm not sure it would be possible to farm without them. Dave and I certainly wouldn't have learned to farm without friends. Friends listen when you complain, they lend you equipment, they share your natural disasters, they help you physically if you need extra workers, and they give you advice.

Once I realized that nothing bad or embarrassing happened when I asked questions, we began to take advantage of the incredible stores of knowledge and experience in the farmers in our community. Our first questions were very basic and not very well defined.

"What should we do with this field?" we asked Howard.

Howard paused and scratched his beard. "One could put oats there."

"How do you plant oats?"

"Well, first one could plow up the alfalfa." Howard paused.

74

"The alfalfa isn't good anymore?" I blurted into the silence.

"One could replant it."

"This year?"

Pause. "No. Alfalfa won't germinate where it's just been growing. That's why you should plant oats this year."

Eventually, the conversation terminated in Howard's offer to plow, plant, and harvest our oats for a share of the crop. I had long since grown impatient with the long pauses and left the negotiations to Dave, who rapidly learned the art of conversational silences.

Edith and I, however, could converse for a long time without any pauses. I called Edith for sheep problems. "Have you ever had a sheep with lumps on its lips?" I asked once.

"Sounds like sore mouth," Edith said cheerfully.

"Is it bad?" I asked.

"It's very contagious. Our entire flock had it once," Edith continued. "I even got it on my hands. The doctor didn't recognize it."

"How do you treat it?"

"Give them soft mash to eat. They'll eventually get over it." Then our conversation would travel to other topics. "How are your fleeces this year?" Edith asked.

"Not as clean as I would like," I grumbled. "Next year I'm going to coat them like you do."

Edith and I both raised wool for handspinners, who are willing to pay premium prices for premium fleeces. So Edith and I kept our pastures clear of thistles and other prickly weeds. We fed our sheep in specially designed feeders so that they wouldn't dribble hay into their own or each other's fleeces. And we went to the extreme of fitting our sheep with canvas or polyester coats to keep their fleeces clean.

When friends see the sheep coats for the first time, they invariably comment on them. "If those coats had numbers on them, you'd think you were at a race track."

"What a great idea," I respond.

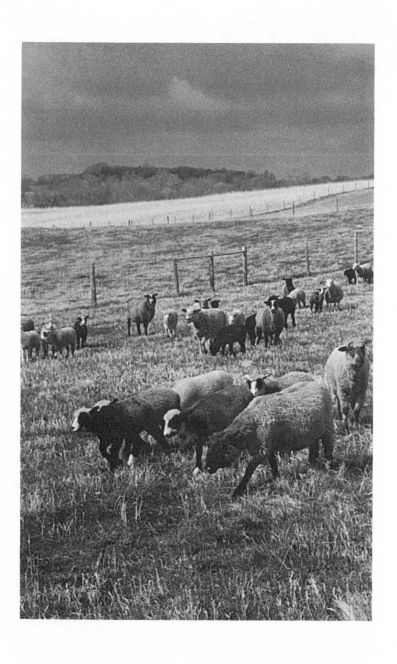

Sheep Racing

logging across the pasture with a bucket of grain and a bucket of supplies, I wondered why I was raising sheep. When I bought my first four lambs, I didn't realize that I'd be lucky if they brought in sixty dollars apiece per year. I'd put a lot of money and a tremendous amount of effort into my sheep operation without any profit. As I weighed alternatives in my mind, sheep racing seemed no more ridiculous than what I was doing now. In my imagination, I built a new industry.

At first glance, sheep are not the obvious race animal. They aren't long-legged and sleek like racehorses. They aren't slender and streamlined like greyhounds. About the only physical characteristics sheep have in common with other race animals is the standard body: one head, one tail, four feet. But, I thought, with selective breeding I could build a stable of tall, sleek race sheep. They would have muscular thighs (after all, we already breed for big legs of lamb) and powerful lungs. They would have the strength and stamina to be winners. Their long fleeces would actually be an advantage. They could be trimmed to any aerodynamically sound shape.

Sheep are excellent runners. They run when a

stranger enters the pasture. They run when you try to catch them. They run when you come to feed them. They run when a dog gets near them.

For the races, we could motivate the sheep to run in one of two ways. A shepherd could chase them around the mile-long track (admittedly hard on the shepherd). Or we could "run" a mechanical ear of corn in front of them—probably the best bet. Shepherds are scarce to begin with, and asking them to chase sheep around a track in front of a crowd would probably bring about the extinction of the breed.

Sheep would also make good steeplechasers. I've seen a ewe clear a three-foot fence to get to her lamb. Rams can easily jump a five-foot fence to reach a ewe in heat. However, the addition of a jockey might really cramp their jumping abilities.

Running ability and motivation won't be the problem. Catching the fancy of the race-going public may be troublesome, however. A racehorse is a high-class, elegant animal. It follows then that people who frequent horse races are high-class, elegant people. A sheep, on the other hand, is neither high-class nor elegant. Cuddly, fluffy, a children's animal. Certainly not something you'd want to risk money on. It would take good advertising to convince the public that they wanted to go to the sheep races.

Good facilities would do much toward that goal. First I'd get the township to surface the road that runs by our farm. Then we'd lay out a big asphalt parking lot—ten or twenty acres of hayfield should be big enough. The racetrack itself would be gaudily tasteful (or is that tastefully gaudy?), with flags flying the colors of each sheep racing that day. The stands would include cheap hard benches for common people and plush boxes, which would rent for thousands of dollars. We'd have lots of boxes. Sheep racing would become chic.

The stables would also be important. If the stables don't look classy, they won't attract classy (rich) sheep owners. The entire operation should exude elegance.

Once we were sure we could attract the racegoers, we'd have to persuade the sheep farmers to change their breeding goals. Instead of breeding for meat and wool, they'd have to breed for speed and stamina. Or perhaps a better strategy would be to persuade that class of well-to-do people who might own racehorses that they should own race sheep instead. After all, sheep are much easier to keep than horses. They are smaller and eat less food. Just think of the savings. The investors would get a much higher return on their investments with sheep than horses.

Sheep are easier to handle than horses. You can't set a horse on its rump with its front legs in the air. Easily done with a sheep (once you catch it). When you've got the sheep in that position, they are completely docile. Horses aren't docile in that position; then again, who's ever seen a horse sitting on its rump? Certainly trainers would be interested in working with an animal that loves to run and is small enough to control easily.

I realize that the standard attributes of a sheep, beyond cute and cuddly, also includes dumb. That is practically slanderous. They are not dumb. They are very single-minded and extremely gregarious. Where one goes, they all go. If the first sheep doesn't want to go where the shepherd directs her, none of the other sheep will go. These traits make the sheep an ideal animal for racing. They'll want to stay close together, making each race very exciting.

There was the idea, fully developed in my mind.

Sheep bred for competition, running at an elegant race-track located in our north pasture. People swarming in the backyard. Cars parked in the hayfield. Our quiet country road a busy thoroughfare.

No!

Some things are worth more than money: solitude, quiet, time, peace of mind.

Dumb Animals

Early on a cool September morning, I found myself back in reality again. The clouds had come down to touch the ground. The air was gray and moist. I walked across the pasture, knee-high alfalfa slipping wetly across my shiny black boots, soaking my jeans.

I didn't mind the wet or the walk. The rains had finally come. It was reassuring to have all this alfalfa to use as pasture. The fall before we were feeding bales of hay by this time. Then we discovered temporary electric fencing. Now when our pastures give out, we set the fences up in the hayfield and extend our grazing season by several weeks. This year we've been moving the sheep around the hayfield. The little clusters of brown and white sheep remain isolated by a bubble of electric fencing, connected to the main pasture by the umbilical cord of the hose from the pump to the water tank.

Autumn is the easy time of the year for shepherds. The lambs are all old enough so they don't get sick. The ewes aren't pregnant and they aren't lactating, so they don't have problems. My only job is to make sure that they have plenty of food and water. Thus the six hundred feet of electric fencing and four hundred feet of garden hose.

Every five days, I moved the sheep to a new pasture. Moving the sheep is an exercise in ovine ("ovine," I quickly learned, means "sheep") intuition. Without it, people can't really get them to move well at all.

We began moving sheep in the typical novice shepherd fashion, running after them, flapping our arms, and barking. The sheep certainly did move. They scattered to all corners of the field. Then we would begin all over again. Eventually we discovered that more people worked better with this pseudodog technique, and we'd move the sheep only when we had guests. A group of six or eight people running around the pasture, flapping their arms and barking was quite a sight. Frequently I'd just watch, calling directions to my barking, flapping crew. "Go north, Laurel! Stop!" "Amber, come back toward me!" "I said north, Dave!" "Paul! Stop!" My crew's inability to follow directions plus the exhausting nature of the technique finally forced us to reassess our routine.

For a while we just left gates open, hoping that all the sheep would eventually work their way into the new pasture. But this was incredibly time consuming and worked poorly. Next I baited the new pasture with a bucket of grain. Fair, of course, found the grain immediately and frequently ate it all before anyone else even walked into the new pasture. Trying to protect the grain from Fair, I stumbled across the sheep-moving technique used by dogless shepherds around the world: enticing them with a bucket of grain.

I walk into the pasture with a bucket of corn. "Hey, ewes," I call, shaking the bucket like a rattle. Fair perks up her ears and begins moving toward me. "Hey, ewes." The sheep around Fair look up. Soon the entire flock is moving in my direction. I head toward the new pasture. They pick up speed. So do I. Just ahead of the thundering herd, I pass through the gate and move as far as possible into the new pasture before the sheep surround me. If I stop too soon, the sheep block the gate, and those in the rear never change pastures. So I have to run while watching over my shoulder until the last sheep is through the gate. Then I dump the corn on the ground and walk nonchalantly back to the gate, trying to get there before the sheep change their minds about where they want to be. It takes the new lambs only two or three moves to recognize the sound of the bucket and my "Hey, ewes." It took me only two or three years to discover the technique. The question does come to mind, Who is the dumb animal on this farm?

When we first got the sheep, moving them was so exhausting that we seldom bothered. But with the advent of temporary electric fencing and insight into ovine intuition, we began moving them weekly. We wade out to the fence line through the high alfalfa, disconnect the battery, and gingerly pull up the first stake. I've never gotten a shock from my fence, so I probably overestimate its strength. But I'm a terrible coward around electric fences.

Dave then dumps a bucket of oats in a corner of the pasture, and all the sheep cluster around him, intent on the oats. We quickly reset one section of fence around them, enclosing them in a very small bubble of fence so that we can reset the rest of the fence around a new section of alfalfa.

Fair, always so intent on her food, shoves her head into the bucket. The handle flops over her ears. After she's finished the last few grains, she raises her head, and the bucket comes, too. Fair is so tame, she stands there waiting for us to remove that funny thing and give her sight again. When Brownie tries the same trick, she panics and dashes blindly around the pasture with a bucket on her head and Dave and me on her heels. We aren't fast enough to catch her or ovine enough to guess which direction she'll go next. Finally we resort to stealth, carefully approaching from two directions and herding her into a corner of the pasture. When she reaches the fence, she panics again, but this time our minds are in sheep mode and our muscles are set. Dave grabs a hind leg as she passes by, and we have her! Maybe some day I'll learn not to set the grain bucket down in the pasture.

Fencing has become a routine chore. Dave and I can pull up and reset six hundred feet of fence and move the waterer, salt feeder, and sheep in two hours. Quite an improvement over my first attempt.

Originally I bought one hundred fifty feet of temporary electric fence to use for a ram pasture. The directions suggested setting it up in an enclosed area, with the electric fence directly in front of a wall or permanent fence so that if the sheep tried to go through, they would learn that they couldn't. I began unrolling the fence in the ram pasture. The temporary electric fencing that we use is called electric netting. It is a large-spaced plastic net with metal wires running through the horizontal strands and extra reinforcing on the vertical strands. Every ten feet, there is a plastic-covered metal post that can be pushed into the ground. One end of the fence is attached to the charger, which runs off of a battery.

I began fencing at noon. Somehow, I had the fence twisted several times before I got it unrolled. This meant that after setting two or three posts, I'd have to untwist the rest of the fence. The rams were very interested and kept coming over to investigate. The instruction manual warned that the sheep shouldn't touch the fence unless it was on so that they would immediately respect it. I tried luring the rams away with corn, but they finished the corn much more quickly than I finished the fence. In fact, I spent almost three hours setting up one hundred fifty feet of fence.

With the fence finally up, I hurriedly hooked the battery to the fence charger and the fence charger to the fence. I was rapidly following the manual step by step. Red wire to the positive pole on the battery, black wire to the negative pole, green wire to the fence, and earth wire to the grounding rod.

I didn't have a grounding rod! I unhooked the wires and patiently began pulling up fence posts. I would have to go to town to get a grounding rod. If the manual said not to let the sheep touch the fence, I wouldn't, but it seemed a terrible waste of time. By now the rams had lost interest in me and the fence, so at least I was able to role the fence up unmolested.

At the hardware store they sold me an eight-foot long copper rod about a centimeter in diameter. I returned home determined to set up the grounding rod, battery, and charger first. The grounding rod would not go into the ground. I reached as high as possible and hung on it. The rod didn't budge. Amber and Laurel hung on it with me. It wouldn't go into the earth far enough to support itself. I was too short to pound on the top of the rod with a hammer. Finally I called Dave at work. I always hate to bother him, and I'd much rather figure things out by myself, but the rams needed new pasture, so I had to get the fence up that day. Dave suggested softening the ground by running water onto it and then making a hole with the hose. It worked beautifully. Fifteen minutes later, I had the grounding rod in place.

Starting at the charger, I began unrolling and resetting fence. I would unroll a few feet and then stop to untangle the posts where they had wormed their way into the netting. This was much worse than the first time. And the rams were again fascinated. They kept trying to eat the shiny black wires. Totally frustrated by now, I rerolled the fence and got the kids. "Keep the rams away from the fence," I told them. "They're not supposed to touch it." With shouts and screams and flapping gestures, Amber and Laurel held the rams at bay for half an hour while I set up the fence. It didn't follow the fence line nearly as well as it had the first time, but I hoped that they would get the idea.

I made the final connections and turned on the charger. The indicator didn't light up, so I checked the connections. Red to positive, black to negative, green to fence, the other black to ground. I turned the fence on. Nothing. The kids and I walked the fence line looking for a tall piece of grass or stick that might discharge it. Nothing. Finally we began taking the fence down again. This time I rolled carefully, keeping the ends of the posts outside the netting.

At 4:57 P.M. I called the fencing company. Fortunately, someone was still working. I explained my problem. The man thought for ten seconds. "It sounds to me," he said, "like you have the ground wire and the wire for the negative pole mixed up."

"How can I tell the difference?" I asked.

"Oh, the ground wire has a label that says 'earth' on it."

I thanked him for his help and headed for the pasture. My ground wire didn't say "earth," I was sure of that, but I would try reversing the black wires.

Not only did my ground wire say "EARTH" in half-inch silver letters; it was also twice the diameter of the other black wire.

The kids and I put up the fence for the last time in half an hour. They distracted the rams while I unrolled the fence and set the posts. Half past five. I flipped the switch on the charger. The indicator light flickered red. The fence was on!

Yes, the fence was on; and I'd put the fence between us and the gate. As the sun sank in the west and the rams learned that electric fencing is not for eating, I boosted the kids over the barbed-wire fence and then climbed over myself, ripping my pants on the dismount.

Days like that really tested my self-confidence. If an intelligent, well-educated person like me couldn't do a simple task in less than five hours, how did under-educated farmers figure things out? And if most farmers had no trouble setting up electric fencing, did I really have any business trying to farm?

Fortunately, the ability to set up fences is not a pre-requisite for fulfilling the winter needs of sheep. They need clean water, good hay, and late in their pregnancies, nice grain.

The winter routines of caring for sheep don't require great amounts of time or effort either. Winter, prelamb-ing winter, is the time to rest up for lambing. Time to prepare oneself mentally and physically for the frantic times of lambing.

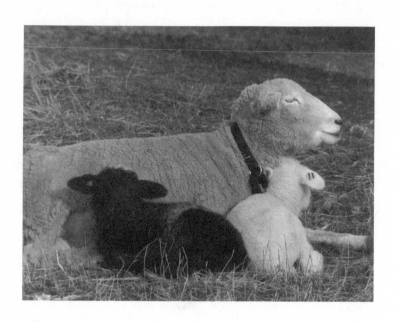

Maternity Ward

Puddles was having trouble. She'd given birth about 7 A.M.; now it was noon, and she still wasn't paying much attention to the lamb. Puddles's sides weren't at all sunken and she kept pawing the ground, trying to make a nest.

Twice I washed my hands, lubricated them, and pushed my fingers over the dark purplish red amnion that bulged out of her vagina. I felt nothing and was afraid to push further. But every time Puddles strained with a contraction, I could tell there was something huge in there trying to get out.

Finally I got Dave. "I think there's another lamb in there. I have to get it out, and I have to do it myself. Just give me emotional support. Tell me I'm doing all right."

For a third time, I washed and lubricated my hands. Then, with Dave holding Puddles's head, I knelt behind her and slid my hand into her vagina. The first thing I felt was a pointed little hoof. I closed my eyes and explored the hoof with my fingers. The flat side and sharp edges were down—it was facing the right direction, so probably the lamb was facing the right direction. My fingers pushed further and found the lamb's nose, then his jaw, and then the eyebrows.

Next I had to decide if the head and hoof were connected. I might be dealing with two lambs tangled together instead of just one. I tried moving my fingers back along the head to the lamb's shoulder, but I ran into the bones of Puddles's pelvis in every direction. This lamb was a tight fit. I pulled my hand back slightly until my fingers found the hoof again. Carefully I explored it. It was only one hoof, with the characteristic split down the middle. I could feel the smooth curves of the top and the flat planes of the bottom. My fingers moved down and sideward. There! Another hoof! Carefully my fingers followed this hoof up the leg to the elbow. Beyond that I couldn't go; pelvic bones again blocked the way.

My fingers returned to the first hoof. Gently I pulled it toward the opening of Puddles's vagina. The leg stretched out, but I still couldn't follow it to the lamb's body.

Taking stock of the situation, I tried to picture in my mind what I was feeling with my fingers. Two hooves, facing in the right direction, one slightly ahead of the other. One head, above and behind the hooves. That was a perfect presentation, the lamb ought to come.

The time for visualization and exploration was over. I had to do something. For the first time since we had bought sheep, I had to help a ewe lamb. As long as I thought of the process in the abstract, I was fine. If I allowed my mind to expand, to think of repercussions, problems, then I started to sweat.

"I'm going to try to help it out," I said to Dave. "I think I can work on its foot." Carefully I pulled again on one leg, fingers slipping over the slick surface. I clamped my fingers tight. This time Puddles's contractions helped, and a small white hoof came into view. "There's a hoof. Where's the other one? Dave, it should be coming." Another contraction, and a white nose peeped out. Protruding from the mouth was a purple tongue, which meant the lamb was in distress. "Dave, it's dying, its tongue is purple." Beginning to panic, I pushed the nose back in and fished again for the second hoof.

"Just relax, Joanie, you're doing fine." Dave's voice calmed me down. I again worked the hooves slowly toward the entrance of Puddles's vagina. First one and then the other. Then I slipped my fingers over the top of the lamb's head, trying to ease it forward. But there just wasn't room for hooves, head, and my fingers at that point. I pulled my hand out and grasped the little white hooves. Pulling out and down, I worked the forelegs out of the ewe. They slid slowly out, first to the ankle, and then the knee. Finally the lamb's nose appeared again. With a hard contraction, Puddles pushed the entire lamb out onto the hay-covered floor. It was a huge ram! And he was fighting hard for life. As I grabbed for a towel, he lifted his head from the ground once, twice, trying to escape from the membrane that still covered his entire body, trying to reach the life-giving air. Hurriedly, I ripped the membrane from his face. Then I picked him up and placed him at his mother's head.

In spite of her exhaustion, Puddles's instincts were sound. She immediately began licking her lamb. First she licked the membrane away from his nose. Then she licked the membrane across his belly and bit through the umbilical cord. Again and again, Puddles's tongue came out, removing the shiny membrane from her lamb's body and drying the amniotic fluid in which he had floated for so long. Finally he was clean and fairly dry. Puddles gave a last few licks as the lamb staggered to his feet and blundered toward his mother's udder, ready to fend for himself.

I looked at Dave and grinned. "That wasn't so hard."

"You did great," he said.

"Thanks for the support. I needed to do that myself, even if you could've done it better."

Dave looked at me. "Delivering babies in the delivery room with several nurses and all the appropriate equipment is a lot different from lambing," he said. "I've never gone searching for a missing leg with my hands."

I grinned. "True. But thanks anyhow. Having you here really helped."

PUDDLES WAS THE first. Polar Bear aborted the next day. She wasn't due for three more weeks. I called the vet because she was acting strangely.

"Have you done a pelvic exam on her?" he asked.

Without pausing to reflect, I lubricated my hand and arm and inserted it into the ewe's uterus. But there was nothing in there. I couldn't find the fetus in the barnyard, either. But I knew she had been pregnant. Her udder was engorged, and she wanted to mother. For several days she'd been sniffing every new baby as if searching for her own.

From then on, I was lambing full time. I didn't have time to worry about Polar Bear and her miscarried baby. Every day brought new adventures. The ewes were lambing two or three at a time. Twins, triplets. Lambs with diarrhea. Ewes with mastitis. Lambs too big to be born easily. Lambs too small to live easily. I got to know the vets better. They came to know me.

I learned to take the ewe's temperature before I called the vet, because he always inquired about it. I also learned to tie a string to my tiny little rectal thermometer so that I could retrieve it when it got lost.

The vets learned that I thought of my sheep as friends—their babies were my babies. I would do what had to be done to keep them well.

Dave left for his eight-day stretch in the emergency room. Laurel, Amber, and I mothered each other, accomplishing what needed to be done and ignoring the rest. Amber learned to wash clothes. Laurel learned to make tacos. I learned to castrate ram lambs by myself and to live without enough sleep, without time for relaxation or even showers.

The barn got fuller, the house got cluttered. The ewes cleaned their babies, my kids cleaned themselves, and I got dirtier.

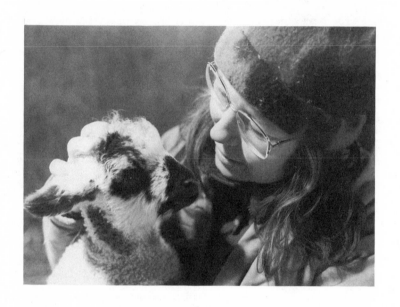

Circles

Clean! For the first time in a week!

For seven days, I had worn sweatpants and a sweat-shirt (usually the same ones) day and night. I climbed out of bed and into my navy sweatsuit at 7 A.M., I struggled out of my sweatsuit and into bed at 10 P.M. Out of bed and into sweatsuit at 1 A.M., out of sweatsuit and into bed at 1:30 A.M. Out of bed and into sweatsuit at 4 A.M., out of sweatsuit and into bed at 4:30.

My hair was like greasy grass. My fingers and finger-nails were grimy with ground-in dirt. It wasn't that I didn't like baths or showers—I literally hadn't had time or energy to take one.

At 2:30 in the afternoon I stripped off the sweatsuit, threw it into the clothes basket and stepped into the shower. How wonderful to be clean! New jeans, a dressy shirt, and fashionable jacket made me feel like a different person. Makeup and a silver bracelet and necklace completed the transformation from shepherdess to wife, mother, me.

The kids and I were going to take a four-hour break from lambing and go to Fargo to have dinner with Dave. I pulled coveralls over my fancy clothes and slipped into boots. One last check in the barn before we left.

Naturally there was a new baby. But more importantly, there was a ewe in trouble. Daffodil was running distractedly in circles with a dry, woolly black-and-white head sticking out of her vagina. The lamb blinked its eyes at me. It was alive! What a terrible presentation! The lamb could die rapidly.

I tackled the ewe, grabbed a front and back leg, and dropped her to the ground. Lying full-length on the ewe, I tried to push the lamb's head back into Daffodil's uterus. No luck.

Edith and Wendy had told me about propping a ewe's hind end up onto a bale of hay to let gravity help slide the lamb back in, but I didn't think there was time to find a bale. I vaguely remembered advice about tying both of the ewe's hind legs to a rope, then passing it across my shoulders. No rope.

I tipped Daffodil onto her back, put her hind legs over my shoulders (occasionally, being short was a real advantage), grabbed her around the waist and lifted. The ewe's hind end rose off the ground. The lamb's head slipped in a little way. Holding the ewe with my stronger arm, I slipped my left hand into Daffodil's vagina alongside of the lamb's head. As my fingers fished for the lamb's leg, my bracelet slid down my arm and banged the lamb's nose. Desperate as I was to save this lamb, I still grinned to myself at the bizarre picture I must have been presenting.

At this point, I thought about calling the veterinarians, but this seemed like a problem I had to solve right now, not wait for someone else to help me.

I could feel the lamb's left shoulder and stretch my fingers back along the long tarsal bones, but I couldn't find a joint. The bone just stretched on forever, way past the tips of my fingers. In my mind I could see the lamb's body packed compactly into that dark, soft, warm uterus, head stretched out into the cold light. A good, big, strong lamb, just not packaged in the right position for birth.

I again tried pushing the lamb's head back into Daffodil's vagina. As I pressed against its nose, the lamb's mouth opened, and it began to suck on my finger. Horrified, I stopped pushing. I could not push this breathing, suckling lamb back into its mother's uterus. But I had to save it. We had already bonded with each other!

The fingers on my left hand didn't "see" as well as the fingers on my right. The shapes they felt behind the head made no sense and had no fingerholds for pulling. And my right arm was aching, shaking, turning to jelly.

I shifted arms, holding the ewe with my left. I slid my right hand along the lamb's neck and shoulder, forcing it further past the constriction of the ewe's cervix. This time I crooked my index finger over his scapula, the large flat bone in the shoulder, and pulled. The shoulder moved. I stretched two fingers out, hooked them into a depression, and pulled again. This time the whole body moved, slowly, minutely, toward me. This was not a good way to pull a lamb. Shoulders weren't meant to slide through the cervix without the passage being eased by the front legs.

Slowly, with continuous pulling, the lamb and my hand eased through the cervix. When the shoulders appeared, I used both hands, searching for depressions or corners in the skeleton, and pulled. Another inch, and I could see the forelegs along its body. Then with a final contraction, Daffodil completed her labor, and a beautiful black and white spotted lamb slid onto the straw.

Had I killed him with my incautious pulling? Had I crushed something important by forcing my hand in beside his head? No! I recognized the shake of his head as the characteristic of a healthy newborn.

Just then Daffodil's second lamb slid onto the straw

next to her brother. This lamb was still wrapped in amnion. As I pulled the membrane away from her face, she lifted her head and then dropped it to the floor. The little white head rose again momentarily and then dropped. This lamb did need help.

I lifted the slippery little body six inches off the floor and then dropped it. The ribs didn't move. I lifted it and dropped it again. Nothing. Grabbing the hind legs at the hocks with my right hand, I gathered the body against my chest and raced out the door. Outside, I swung the lamb up in a semicircle to directly over my head, and then pulled it down into my arms. I checked the ribs for signs of breathing and repeated the procedure. It sounds like rough treatment, but the swings allow gravity to expand and contract the lungs. Usually that's enough to start the lamb breathing. For Daffodil's second baby, the second swing brought shuddering gasps and then breathing. Relaxing, I returned the lamb to her mother for a thorough licking and bonding.

Daffodil's third lamb didn't even try to lift his head. No amount of swinging started his lungs working. I had lost another baby. My self-confidence began to drain away. If I'd called the vet, could I have saved Daffodil's third baby? If I'd found Daffodil sooner, would her third baby still have been alive? If I had lived in the barn during lambing, I might have saved that lamb.

But my family needed me, too. Everything was a compromise. Now that I finally know enough to care well for my sheep, I realize that knowledge isn't enough. My commitments to my family also restrict what I can do for my sheep. There just wasn't time to do everything, be there all the time.

I took stock. My new jeans were soaked with amniotic fluid. My silver necklace lay broken on the ground.

My hand and bracelet were bloody. A dead lamb lay on the floor. But I had two live lambs and a healthy mother. Perhaps a good enough trade.

I installed Daffodil and her spotted lambs in a pen, started the lambs nursing, fed and watered Daffodil, and headed back to the house. Time for another shower!

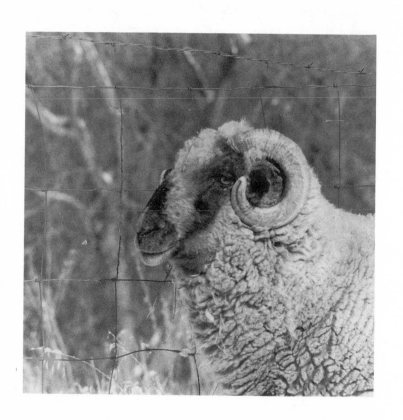

Barbed Wire

Lambing is definitely a shepherdess's most time-consuming activity. It also uses the most emotional energy. But summer's the time when we expend the most physical energy on the sheep. In the summer, we put up hay. In the summer, we fence pasture—digging post-holes, stretching out thousands of feet of barbed wire, and nailing it to the posts. In the summer, we clean up pastures, kill thistles, fix gates, straighten posts, and clean up the patches of barbed wire that have sprung up over the past year.

Our barbed wire harvest runs for some time. For the last hundred years, farmers on our place had planted most of the pastures and wood to barbed wire. Although this appears to have been done in a random manner, the wire was well planted and had flourished. But I raise sheep, and sheep do not coexist well with this particular type of barbed wire. So I decided to reap all the old woven and barbed wire.

It is incredible the way that stuff grows. The roots run for yards underground—or, as it prefers, under rock piles, perhaps because of the excellent aeration. Barbed wire grows amazingly rapidly. I once left a partial roll in my pasture, and several weeks later it had taken root. At this young stage, barbed wire is aggressively carnivorous; it actually reaches out to bite. I've never found any skeletons entangled in the rolls of barbed wire, so perhaps it doesn't actually consume humans but just tastes them. Prevention is the only reasonable solution. A heavy long-sleeved shirt, jeans, and leather gloves improve your chances of surviving harvest unscathed.

Barbed wire also reproduces well. Many of the cuttings we leave lying around during harvest seem to grow into new long healthy wires by morning. This reproductive capability can be a problem when you are fencing. You absolutely must pick up any stray ends of wire that are cut from the fence or the main roll. If given a chance to reproduce, they can be deadly to sheep, machinery, and people careless enough to sit, kneel, walk, or lean on them.

Barbed and woven wire both come in several varieties other than the two-barbed versus four or twelve-inch spacing versus six specified by manufacturers. The most common variety of barbed wire is the creeper. Most of the trees along the edges of our old pasture are slowly being strangled by Virginia creeper and barbed wire, a lethal combination of clinging vines. We've found that this variety of wire is best harvested with a hacksaw and wire cutters. After cutting, the wire can be carefully untangled from the tree.

The second most common variety of barbed wire is heavy on roots and sparse on stems. Not only do the roots grow hundreds of times longer than the stems; there may actually be two separate roots emerging from both ends of a short horizontal length of stem. Although this variety can be harvested by hand if the wire is not yet well rooted, the most reliable method entails looping a chain around the horizontal stem, fastening the chain to the bumper of a pickup truck, and driving away.

The most common variety of woven wire is the dense mat, which is found immediately above or immediately below ground. This type is most often rust colored, although occasionally the silver galvanized cultivar is seen. The mat type of woven wire is usually reaped with a shovel. Pulling the mat with a pickup truck improves the yield and speed of harvest. If this variety is well rooted, a tractor or pickup is essential.

Another growth pattern for woven wire is the large roll, which is usually intimately associated with a clump of trees. The trees invariably need to be cut down to completely disengage the wire. Unfortunately, a chainsaw cannot be used, since the wire wraps the tree in the only place where it is possible to make a cut. The large roll of woven wire is best harvested by first cutting an area of wire with a hacksaw, then cutting the tree down with a handsaw. You might think that merely cutting the wires would do the job, but that is the secret of the large-roll variety: there are simply too many wires to cut them all. Once the tree is down, you can haul the whole mess away. Frequently you must cut down two or three trees before you can harvest a particular roll of wire.

With the quantity of ripe wire on our property and the presence of several varieties of both woven and barbed wire, I had great hopes for our harvest. New woven wire was selling for $58 per hundredweight, considerably more than the approximately $8 we'll get for our barley. But there doesn't seem to be a very good market for vintage woven wire. The shepherds, who have traditionally used woven wire to keep the sheep in the pastures and the predators out, are going out of business.

The market for used barbed wire among farmers is even worse. No one seems to have the time or the patience to untangle and straighten vintage wire. Although collectors pay good money for ridiculously small pieces of barbed wire, I can't even give mine away. It is too common. Finally, in desperation, I called the sanitation service in town and filled a huge dumpster three times. I had to pay them to haul my harvest away.

I also had to pay Dave's brother Paul to help me with the harvest. We worked two entire days, cutting and gathering the barbed and woven wire. The wire dulled my wire cutters, a handsaw, and a hacksaw blade. I ruined a good pair of leather gloves and am nursing numerous holes in my body.

Despite the obvious affinity barbed wire has for my land, I realize that I could never raise it as a cash crop. The only people who should even think about its economic potential are tool manufacturers, sanitation companies, and Paul.

Paul, like most of our friends, enjoys the sheep in a remote sort of way. He would rather be remote from them when we need to work them. Everyone seems to be remote—as in gone—when I have troubles with the sheep.

Trouble

Bosho the ram was out! We put him in a covered pickup in the evening so that I could take him to Edith's farm to do his duty as a stud in the morning. Dave tied the back window shut with baling twine. Come morning, one hour after Dave left for a week at work and the girls left for school, I found the truck empty.

Fortunately, we still had some ewes in heat. And sure enough, Bosho was pacing the fence line as close to the ewes as he could get.

I caught him easily. He ignored me when I approached him and grabbed him around the neck. I couldn't move him. I pulled and pushed as hard as I could. He wasn't even affected by my presence. I slipped a grain bucket over his head and tried to lead him. Nothing. Bosho wouldn't budge away from the fence. The only result of our tug-of-war was my sore feet and muddy shoes from his repeatedly stepping on me. At this point I really wished he was still wearing his marking harness with its bright orange crayon. Each ram had his own harness holding a marking crayon on his chest. I could tell which ewes had been bred with which ram by the color of the crayon marks on their rumps. I already had enough ewes marked with Bosho's distinctive orange crayon. Now it was Solomon's turn in with my ewes and Bosho's turn with Edith's. Even if the harness hadn't been designed to help shepherdesses drag stubborn rams around, it would have been a big help.

Only the day before, we had moved the sheep successfully around the backyard. I figured Bosho would follow the ewes anywhere, so I let them out of the pasture now. Bosho eagerly followed the ewes, but they wouldn't follow me.

The day before, there had been four of us herding sheep. This time there was only me. I was no threat. The grass and flowers in the backyard were much more interesting than the bucket of grain I was carrying.

"Hey ewes," I called, "hey ewes." I rattled the corn in the bucket over and over again. Brownie had begun browsing on my yellow roses, and the first group of sheep was rounding the corner of the house heading away from me. Panic was flickering in my brain when Fair looked up. Good old fat Fair, always interested in the bucket. She started toward me, and one or two of the others glanced in my direction. They paused. Cocoa started after Fair, who was now running. As the lead sheep picked up speed, the rest of the flock gradually changed its orientation. By the time I walked through the gate, they were all behind me and heading for the pasture. By the time I rounded the corner of the barn, running hard, they were all through the gate and in the pasture, also running hard.

I ran down the slope, around the last corner, and into the barn. Everyone plowed into the barn behind me, propelled by greed or habit. Habit also helped me squeeze them into the corner by the loading ramp using several hog panels. They circled behind the panels, not independent enough to break through. Not smart enough to realize that as long as I hadn't tied the panels in place, they weren't actually a barrier.

Bosho was still ardently pursuing his chosen ewe round and round the pen, nose up in the air, lips wrinkled back in a particularly rammy expression. When he passed the loading ramp, I threw myself against him. I must have taken him by surprise. When he realized that his ewe was no longer in front of him, he dug in his heels and tried to turn around, but we were already halfway up the ramp. I braced myself against the walls of the ramp to keep him from going back down. With surprisingly little brute strength, I was able to encourage him on up the ramp and into the truck. I tied the back window shut with three pieces of twine and backed the truck up against the barn. Even if he broke the twine, he wouldn't be able to force the window open more than six inches. He would be safe until I was ready to leave.

I dismantled the pen and let the ewes out of the barn. They surged into the barnyard and straight toward the still-open gate.

"Nooo!" With an agonized burst of speed, screeching at the top of my lungs, I arrived at the gate just in front of the lead ewe. Either desperation lent me speed, or my screeching slowed them down. At any rate, forty-five minutes after I looked into my empty truck, Bosho was on his way to a new harem and the ewes were once again safe in their pasture.

Of course, no pasture was really impregnable during breeding. When I returned from Edith's, the ewes were grazing in the garden again. And somehow, three rams I wasn't using for breeding this year had joined them.

I knew I wouldn't be able to sort four rams from forty sheep all by myself, so I waited for the girls to come home from school. Even with their help, the struggle was herculean.

We started with a bucket of corn. Fair and Solomon, my breeding ram, both believed my con job and followed me. Amber and Laurel hassled the stragglers. We moved all the sheep back into the barnyard. I shut the gate. The bar was broken and Solomon's head was bloody. He had obviously wanted to get out very badly.

Solomon followed his ewes into the barn for a drink of water. We pulled the doors shut. But the majority of the ewes and three ram lambs—number 42, a white; 27, a brown; and the spotted number 1—were still in the pasture.

I dumped a pile of corn on the ground and stood quietly while the hungry sheep gathered around. The brown ram lamb was canny. I stood quietly beside the grain pile for a long time. He came to eat easily, but every time my body moved the least little bit, he was off again. I launched myself at him time after time, only to land face-first in the dirt. Amber and Laurel cheered me after each landing but couldn't really help. Finally, more through luck than skill, I grabbed a handful of fleece. We dragged him to the fence, and the girls held him against it. Then I wrapped a piece of baling twine around his chest and dragged him to the ram pasture.

Number 42, the white ram, was the real problem. He was in heaven! Head stretched forward, nose wrinkled, lips pulled back, tongue hanging out. He darted from ewe to ewe, sniffing each one. He was like a dirty-minded little boy. I was infuriated. That was not the ram I wanted to father next spring's lambs. After half an hour of chasing him around the pasture, we gave up. We could not separate him from the ewes he had claimed. Finally we chased him and his two ewes into a separate pasture and slammed the gate.

Only one uninvited ram was left in the breeding pasture. I sprinkled corn all along the fence line. When all the animals lined up at the fence to eat, I grabbed handfuls of number 1's brown-and-white fleece through the fence. Fortunately, the sheep were crowded so closely that he couldn't escape. I pried the bottom of the fence up with one foot. Then I shifted my grip one hand at a time to his legs. Amber and Laurel pushed while I pulled him under the fence.

Kneeling astride him, I wrapped the twine harness across his chest, under one leg and over his shoulders. With a good grip on the harness, I stood up. We bolted out the gate.

He started circling around me, an arm's length away, at full speed. Once, twice, three times.

My hand was in agony, my fingers were turning blue. My feet were unsteady, and the world was spinning. Wrenching my hand from the harness, I dropped to my knees. Ram number 1 darted off—fortunately, away from the ewe pasture.

I staggered to my feet. The girls pushed the gate shut and slid what was left of the bar into the hole in the fence post. I tied the gate shut with three pieces of twine. Maybe it would look solid, and Solomon wouldn't try to take it down.

Twenty-four hours later, the sheep were in the garden again. They obviously wanted more interesting food than the dried, yellow-brown grass left in the home pasture. Solomon was not at all fooled by my baling-twine illusions.

I filled my bucket with corn and approached Solomon. When he stuck his head in the bucket, I grabbed his harness with its yellow crayon and steered him toward the barn. He would not escape again. The concrete block barn had steel doors. Even Solomon could not break them down. After I sorted out the ram lambs, I could feed the ewes and Solomon and stop worrying about breakouts.

With Solomon out of trouble, I began working on the ram lambs again. To my surprise, I cornered both of the loose lambs quite easily. The girls sat on the rams while I drove the pickup down to the pasture. I had planned for these lambs to go to market sooner or later. They'd caused enough trouble that they were going sooner.

I didn't grieve when I delivered those three lambs to the butcher.

Gates

Fall is not normally a time of troubles. The ewes are happy, with plenty of pasture. The rams are busy with the ewes. The girls are busy back in school. So I can restart my volunteer work, at the school, at church, and in Camp Fire. With Amber and Laurel gone most of the day, I find time for thinking, assessing, being aware of the world around me.

Half past five on a cold October morning. I was leaving in fifteen minutes for an all-day Camp Fire workshop, and the sheep had to have fresh pasture. So I had fifteen minutes to move them, shower, and put on respectable Camp Fire clothes.

I was wearing a down parka. The air was cold, the sky was black, and the stars were intense pinpricks of light. It was like a winter night, almost like lambing. I didn't have a flashlight. I assumed that it would be light out.

The first gate was just a sliding bar; it opened easily. The second gate was a sliding bar and a piece of baling twine tied in a square knot or maybe a granny. But my fingers untied it automatically. I've tied and untied that kind of knot so many times, I can do it in the dark with ice-cold fingers. I climbed the third gate, as I'd never get all the twisted ends of wire untwisted in the short time

I'd allowed myself. The fourth gate was also shut with twisted wire, but I had to open this one to let the sheep through. I felt down the edge of the gate, stopping to untangle each horizontal wire from the vertical fence wire. Two, three, five wires untangled. I pulled the gate open and called the sheep. "Hey ewes."

Not a sound, no one moved. I could see them, vague white mounds sleeping soundly under the trees in the corner of the pasture, like huge rocks nestled deep in the pasture soil. They were secure in their knowledge that it was still night and there was no good reason for them to get up and move. A coyote or dog would have been a good reason. But their shepherdess was not a threat, so they didn't budge. Oh well, they'd find the open gate when the sun rose.

I let myself out the gate on the far side of the pasture. My eyes had adjusted to the night so well that I could see the hook and chain to unlatch them. I hiked across the field, enjoying the brisk wind, the trees looming black against the night sky, the familiar constellations —Cassiopeia, the Big Dipper. I turned down the driveway toward the house. Suddenly, I was blind again. The light at the back door shone into my eyes and overwhelmed my night vision. The night was again a tunnel of blackness, and I hurried to get inside.

The Camp Fire workshop was a training session for leaders. We had sessions on bookkeeping, planning the Camp Fire year, and craft ideas. My record keeping was abysmal. I learned a lot. Fibers were the focus in crafts for the year. I taught twenty other leaders how to make "God's eyes," simple off-loom weavings using two sticks and several colors of yarn. Another leader demonstrated wrapped yarn baskets. I was entranced—another fiber art to learn.

The keynote speaker was a child psychologist. She talked about different kinds of families and how to help kids in dysfunctional families. This woman seemed to be in her late thirties, about my age. She had a doctorate in psychology. If I hadn't stayed home to take care of my kids, I mused to myself, I might have been in her position now, delivering a keynote address to some group somewhere.

After ten years of mothering, I had lost most of my knowledge in biochemistry. No way could I speak as an expert now. I couldn't remember the Michaelis-Menton equation or how to differentiate the three kinds of RNA. Even the basics were becoming fuzzy. If I needed science information, I had to look it up. It wasn't stored in my head anymore.

DURING THE TWO-HOUR drive to my workshop, I had reassessed myself and the sheep. The blindness of this morning has stretched back through my shepherdessing. It was psychological rather than physiological, but still effective. My fear of sounding stupid handicapped me for so long. When Roses' baby died, it didn't occur to me to call the veterinarian. My books didn't mention calling the vet for sick lambs. I couldn't imagine bothering Dr. Hexum in the middle of the night. I couldn't ask for help from anyone but Dave, who knew how dumb I was when it came to sheep.

After Spot died of the worm infestation, I began taking fecal samples to the vet frequently. The death of a sheep I knew was much worse than the death of a lamb. I had failed in my responsibility to Spot. I hadn't paid close enough attention to her. I hadn't called the vet when I'd realized she was sick. I had decided to observe her a little bit longer. I'd been afraid to show my ignorance. Afraid to stand out from the other farmers. Afraid to be dependent on anyone but Dave and myself.

Fear was a barrier inside of me that I couldn't unlock or untangle. Each successive death made the barrier more tangled but also increased the pressure to get through that gate.

I wasn't afraid to learn at my Camp Fire workshop. I accepted corrections for stupid mistakes in bookkeeping as easily as I corrected other women when they had problems with their "God's eyes." I had learned as a graduate student, painfully at times. I remembered asking at least one incredibly stupid question at a national conference on cancer research. Why didn't I fear appearing stupid in those situations?

When I'd found Daffodil with a lamb's head sticking out of her vagina, several of the wires closing my internal gates had untangled. Daffodil was a friend of mine, a wonderful mother with a beautiful, distinctive fleece. I couldn't lose her. As I'd worked to deliver her baby, I'd considered calling the vet. I had saved her myself. That had increased my self-confidence. But I had also accepted the idea of asking for help. The gates were beginning to open.

I was also learning to see the sheep in general as farm animals rather than pets. I didn't have the emotional resilience necessary to mourn each individual lamb when I took them to market. I still thanked them, but I couldn't mourn them. I had come to accept that planned death as well as unplanned death was part of being a shepherd.

I knew that sometimes I needed to cause the lambs pain to keep them healthy. But now I could do the painful medical procedures well, causing the least amount of physical and emotional pain to the lambs and myself.

I was confident in myself. I performed many functions, from opening gates to castrating lambs, by rote, doing casually what was once unimaginable. And I was reaching the point were I had knowledge to share.

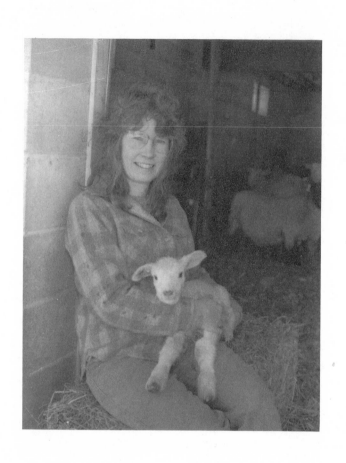

The Mother-Daughter Bond

Knowledge to share. Experiences to share.

The sheep started lambing the day Dave left for his seven-day stretch of work, and Mom and Dad came to help.

Mom, a short, white-haired seventy-year-old lady in Dave's size forty long bloody brown coveralls sat on an overturned bucket in the barn. The golden glow of a hundred-watt bulb threw the wrinkles of her face into relief.

Mom held lamb after lamb cradled in her arms.

First we castrated them. "Why do you have to castrate them?" Mom asked.

"Everyone says they cause too much trouble in the feedlot if they aren't castrated," I explained. "Feedlot owners don't want to have to separate male from female lambs. They want it as easy as possible." I grimaced. "I've read that uncastrated lambs gain lean weight faster than wethers, but the stockyards pay less for rams. So I've never taken the risk of not castrating the rams."

"Maybe they gain weight better because they don't get hurt," Mom said.

"I've thought that, too. Some year I won't castrate them. But not this year."

Mom sat each ram lamb in her lap, facing away from her. Then she pulled his hind legs up and against his chest, exposing his scrotum. I slid the little green rubber rings over the four prongs of the elastrator. I squeezed the handle and the prongs separated, stretching the ring. I slid the ring down over his scrotum and pressed into his belly with my finger and thumb until his testicles moved out into his scrotum. Then, still pressing in, I released the elastrator. The rubber ring contracted around his scrotum. I felt to be sure there were two little round testicles in there, and then I slipped the prongs out from under the ring as quickly as possible. This always seemed to hurt the lambs, and they struggled. When the lambs are in pain, they bleat. Then their mothers look over the edge of the pen with their big brown eyes and baaa worriedly. My mother held on tightly.

Mom and I castrated about a dozen lambs in the group pen that afternoon. They looked awful, lying there on their sides, like a whole pen full of dead lambs. But two hours later when we went to check on the ewes, all the lambs were up and running around.

I think Dave shuts his eyes when we castrate. I know Mom shuts hers when we cut off tails.

After castration, we tagged each lamb in the ear, and then we cut off their tails. "Why do you use ear tags?" Mom asked.

"I need them for my breeding program," I explained. "When you have more than four sheep, you need some way to recognize them. The tags help me to keep track of which sheep had the nicest fleeces, who had the most babies, whose babies gained weight fastest, and who were the best mothers."

The plastic ear tags fit into a punch-type applicator. The applicator makes tagging easy on the lamb and the shepherd. I fit the tag into the applicator, slip the applicator over the ear, and squeeze. The applicator punches a hole in the ear and inserts the tag all in one motion. It takes a while for the lambs to grow into their tags. They seem so big at first. The tagged ear droops. Females are tagged in the left ear, males in the right. Boys have all the rights, that's how we remember. Of course, on the farm, boys also go to market, so they can keep their rights.

Tail docking is the hardest chore for me—and the most dangerous one for the lamb. "So why do you cut off their tails?" Mom asked. "They're so cute with their long wiggling tails."

"Yeah, but if they get diarrhea, the feces get on their tails. Then flies lay their eggs in the feces," I said. "Then the eggs hatch and the maggots feed on the lamb."

Mom wrinkled her nose. "In Laurel's words, 'That's gross!'"

I nodded. "Really gross! I've only had maggots in a lamb once, and I never want to see them again. So we have to dock their tails, no matter how hard it is."

Mom held the lamb tightly in her lap, controlling all four feet. First I squeezed the tail with a Burdizo, a pair of heavy specialty pliers. The Burdizo crushes the bone that runs through the tail and hopefully crushes the blood vessels also. Crushed vessels bleed less than cleanly cut vessels, and bleeding is definitely a problem with docking. With a freshly sharpened knife I cut off the tail. I squirted blood stop powder on the stub, pocketed the tail piece for disposal, and waited patiently for an undetermined amount of time for the blood to clot.

"How long do you wait?" Mom asked.

"I don't know. I just wait," I explained. "Sometimes I wait too long, and they bleed. Sometimes I don't wait long enough, and they bleed. And sometimes I wait just the right amount of time, and they don't bleed."

I removed the Burdizo from the lamb's tail, and blood

spurted onto Mom's coveralls. She patiently squeezed the tail stub with the corner of a bloody towel. This was the fourth lamb out of five whose tail had bled. "You don't very often wait the right amount of time, do you?" she said.

"I'm still trying to figure out what the right amount of time is. The thing that worries me is that it might have nothing to do with time, and then I have no idea how to keep them from bleeding."

After a few minutes, the bleeding stopped. I returned the lamb to his mother while my mother noted the lamb's number and sex in the records. Before picking up the next lamb, I checked the lambs we'd already done. The males were all lying down, the females were all happily nursing, and no one's tail was bleeding. I picked up the sixth lamb of the day and started back toward the light.

Mom smiled up at me from her bucket. What a wonderful thing it is to share the most exciting time of the year with my mother. For all of my life she has given to me, taught me wonder and curiosity and joy. Now I have something to share with her. Through my sheep I can feed her wonder, satisfy her curiosity, share with her my joy.

Nutmeg

At the beginning of lambing that year, I told Dad that I wasn't afraid of lambing anymore. I had experienced all the problems there were, and lambing was going to be easy—all joy!

The first day that Nutmeg didn't come to the feeders, I figured she was ready to lamb. I urged her up, and she walked across the barn. Nothing to worry about. Twenty-four hours later, she hadn't lambed, and she wouldn't get up. I took her temperature—normal. I ran my hand across her back, and the skin rippled and twitched—not normal. I examined her mouth and nostrils. Tiny white bubbles were collecting at the edges of her nostrils—definitely not normal.

Nutmeg didn't fight me. From a sheep whose normal behavior around people is to stay as far away as possible, this was frightening in itself.

I got out my sheep books and read up on milk fever and pregnancy toxemia, or, in veterinary terms, calcium deficiency and ketosis. The diseases were both described fuzzily in my books. I read the symptoms and guessed milk fever. At 10 A.M. I gave Nutmeg 120 cc of calcium D gluconate subcutaneously in twenty different sites all over her back. By now, subcutaneous injections had become easy to give. I pulled up a tent of skin, slipped the needle into that space, and injected the drug. Twenty injections was tedious, but Nutmeg didn't even flinch.

Six hours later I repeated the treatment. By 4:30, she still hadn't improved, so I called the vet.

"Have you checked for ketones in the urine?" Dr. Hexum asked. I hadn't thought of it. I drove to the clinic to get test strips.

"What do I do if the urine shows ketones?" I asked.

"Give her one cup of corn syrup every four hours, orally."

With sheep, getting a urine sample is supposed to be easy—you hold their mouth and nose closed and they urinate—automatically. Carefully I positioned the test strip, a two-inch by one-quarter-inch strip of plastic, under Nutmeg's vulva. When urine hit the strip, it would change color, depending on the amount of ketones in the urine. Peach meant no ketones. Blue meant too many.

Then I moved to Nutmeg's head, clamped one hand around her mouth and pressed her nostrils shut with the other. Nutmeg moved her head back and forth, trying to dislodge my hands, but she didn't fight me. After what seemed like ages, I checked the keto strip—the color wasn't peach or blue. It hadn't changed at all. In fact, the strip was still dry. I wiped it across her vulva, hoping that the urine had missed the strip—still dry. I repositioned the keto strip in the straw, trying to figure out exactly where the urine would come out and where it would run to. Then I held her mouth and nose shut for two ages. The strip was still dry.

I pondered my problem. The calcium hadn't worked. Both the ewe and her lambs could die if she lay there much longer. I couldn't get a urine sample. The corn syrup wouldn't hurt, and it might help. I ran to the house, took off my boots, found the syrup and a measuring cup, put my boots on, and ran back to the barn.

I poured the corn syrup into a yellow plastic one-cup measure. It was cold in the barn, probably about ten degrees Fahrenheit. The syrup poured slowly. I knelt over Nutmeg's shoulders, my legs on either side of her head. Her straight black horns, dangerous when she was healthy, made good handles in her lethargy. I pried open her mouth and poured in some syrup. She moved her head, and the syrup dribbled down her neck.

I poured again. After a tablespoon or so, it overflowed out of the corner of her mouth and down my sleeve. I pulled her head back against my chest, tipped her mouth up, and poured again, careful not to overwhelm her swallowing reflex and get syrup in her lungs. As I leaned forward, my hair trailed into the half-empty syrup cup. When I straightened, my hair dragged syrup across Nutmeg's face and then stuck to my barn coveralls.

I poured again. Nutmeg's tongue had finally gotten into the exercise. As fast as I poured syrup in the side of her mouth she pushed it back out the front of her mouth. Finally the cup was empty, and there was corn syrup everywhere. Nutmeg looked like her head had been dipped in sugar. Straw was sticking to both of us, head, arms, shoulders. I had no idea how much of the syrup was actually inside her. And I had to repeat this at midnight. Horrors!

The midnight feeding was easier. I warmed the syrup in the microwave, poured it into a pop bottle, and carried it to the barn inside my coveralls. I wedged the bottle into the back corner of her mouth, and Nutmeg drank most of the syrup.

By morning she was no better. The vet, Dr. Magnusson this time, told me corn syrup would probably not work. "Did you test for ketones?" he asked.

I explained that I hadn't been able to get a sample. "She hasn't had anything to drink for three days," I said.

He suggested that I give her an electrolyte solution by gavage—that is, through a tube directly into her stomach. It sounded awful and probably impossible, but I guessed that I could do it.

"Without the test we can't know for sure," Dr. Magnusson said. "But she probably has ketosis. You need to give her dextrose IP."

IP, or intraperitoneal injections, really frightened me. I had to carefully push a hypodermic needle into an invisible triangle on the sheep's back formed by her ribs, backbone, and pelvic girdle. If I pushed too hard or in the wrong place, I might put the needle and the dextrose into an organ instead of into the intraperitoneal space. If I moved the needle sideways once it was in the peritoneum, I might slice a hole in the stomach or intestines. A scary procedure! And of course Dave was at work for four more days. Nothing could wait for four days during lambing—except housework and laundry.

I figured that Nutmeg felt bad enough so that I could do just about anything to her. I hung the gavage bag from the ceiling of the barn with a piece of baling twine. Then I straddled Nutmeg's shoulder, pulled her head back to my chest, and tried to slide a half-inch diameter piece of plastic tubing down her throat.

She didn't feel that badly after all. I couldn't even get it into her mouth. As soon as I pushed the tubing into the side of her mouth, where there were no teeth, Nutmeg's thick black tongue pushed the tubing up to her teeth, and she began to chew it. By the time I had retrieved the tube, the first two inches were covered with tiny holes.

I cut off the end of the tube and tried again. This time, I held Nutmeg's mouth shut so she couldn't chew. The tube moved down easily.

Next I had to be sure that I slid the tube into her stomach and not her lungs. I pushed slowly, trying to keep it toward the back of her throat, listening carefully for a cough or a gurgle, which would mean the tube was positioned incorrectly.

Nutmeg coughed. I jerked the tube back to get it out of her lungs and pulled it out of her mouth entirely.

I began again. Finally eighteen inches of the tube had disappeared into Nutmeg's mouth. I listened carefully at the free end of the tube. No breathing sounds. It should be in her stomach. I attached the tube to the gavage bag and let two quarts of electrolytes flow slowly down the tube into Nutmeg's mouth and hopefully into her stomach. Nutmeg chewed the whole time I was removing the tube. The entire tube was perforated. I'd have to buy a new tube for her 10 P.M. feeding.

The intraperitoneal injection was easier to accomplish than the gavage feeding. But my hands shook as I pushed the needle slowly through the skin and muscle. I was so frightened of doing some internal damage that I almost couldn't do the work. But I knew she'd die if she didn't get the dextrose.

By evening, Nutmeg was worse. She wasn't interested in the buckets of food and water I had left in her pen. She didn't look alert anymore. She lay with her head on the ground, eyes closed. Still pregnant, still breathing, but not at all healthy. I called the clinic again. Dr. Weckwerth said, "You'll need to induce her. Come in and pick up the drug."

I gave Nutmeg the hormones to induce labor at 5:30 P.M. At 10 P.M. I repeated the dextrose and the electrolytes. When I checked the barn at 1 A.M., there had been no change. Nutmeg looked like a dying dragon. Her black horned head lay on the golden straw in a circle of lamplight. Her dark pregnant body faded into the blackness of the barn. She wasn't one of my best sheep: her fleece was coarse, and she was wild and unfriendly. But I put so much effort into her, she became important to me, and I didn't want her to die.

I repeated the electrolytes and dextrose at 10 A.M. and called the vets. I could never tell over the phone which vet I was talking to, so I always gave a complete history of Nutmeg's problem. At this point I didn't care if they thought I was dumb, I just wanted her to get better. "My ewe is still down," I concluded. "She doesn't seem to be in labor yet."

"The hormone takes twenty-four to thirty-six hours to work," Dr. Magnusson said. "Just keep giving her the electrolytes and dextrose. Every three hours. You might try adding an antibiotic to the dextrose to keep her from getting an infection."

By midnight, Nutmeg's belly was hard—she was definitely in labor. But I never saw any contractions. Her belly just got hard and stayed that way.

When I checked the sheep at 6 A.M., there was a large white lamb halfway out of Nutmeg's uterus. I slowly pulled it the rest of the way and set it in front of Nutmeg. She immediately started making mothering sounds and licked it clean. The lamb was strong and was soon butting purposefully at Nutmeg.

Nutmeg tried to get up repeatedly but didn't have enough strength. So I rolled her onto her side and milked some colostrum into a bottle to feed the lamb.

The lamb, Walnut, thrived. She sucked eagerly on the bottle, climbed all over her mother's prone body, and slept curled beside her, with her head on her mother's leg.

Nutmeg didn't eat. She didn't stand. I shifted from IP dextrose to oral propylene glycol and continued with electrolytes given by gavage. As long as she wouldn't eat or drink, I had to find a way to get calories and water into her. I tried to force her to stand every time I went to the barn. When Dave came home, he lifted her and supported her for a few minutes every day.

One week later, Nutmeg began crawling across her pen to reach grain and water. She reached forward with her front legs and dragged her body, trying to push with her hind legs. Nutmeg looked even more like an injured dragon when she moved. But now I knew she was getting better.

One month after she'd first gone down, I opened the big barn door by Nutmeg's pen. As usual, I hoisted her to her feet. Walnut bounded out into the beckoning sunlight. "Maaa," Nutmeg bleated. "Baaa," Walnut responded. Nutmeg took three staggering steps and joined her daughter in the sunshine.

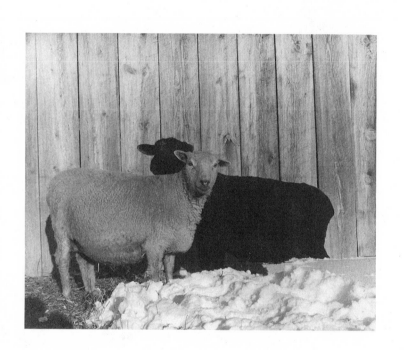

Dying

Walnut was the fourth bottle lamb that year. With that many, I wasn't likely to bond with any of them.

Then Sprinkle lambed. Both lambs, which I catalogued as numbers 52 and 53, were cold when we found them. I don't know if Sprinkle had a hard labor or if she didn't have much milk or if we just weren't checking the barn often enough. We were so tired by then. Dave warmed them when he found them and got them nursing.

By noon the next day, they both looked cold and hungry again. They stood all hunched up and shivering. 52's temperature was only 98 degrees, way below a normal of 103 degrees for sheep. I grabbed both lambs and jugged them, lowering the heat lamp to give them some warmth. Then I gave them warm colostrum. The colostrum might not do any good. They were more than twenty-four hours old and had probably had other food in their stomachs. Once the lining of the stomach has been exposed to other proteins, it stops absorbing immunoglobulins, the disease-fighting ingredient in colostrum that is so important to all baby animals. Some babies die without colostrum. God, I hoped these lambs had nursed enough in the last twenty-four hours to get some of their mother's colostrum.

I could feel myself tightening up. In my head I started running through diseases, symptoms, and cures. Nothing made sense. 52's temperature did not rise. I took him into the house to warm him in the kitchen sink. 52 fit nicely in the sink. His head rested on a corner. The rest of his body floated just below the surface of the water. Bubbles of air caught in his wool slowly worked their way out and rose to the surface of the water. Yellow bits of straw floated around him. He didn't even fight to get out, just lay there with his eyes shut.

I cradled his body in my hands, moving him gently through the warm water. I was afraid to leave him alone, afraid his head would slip beneath the surface and he'd drown, too weak to stand and save himself. One half hour and three unanswered phone calls later, I lifted him out of the sink and laid him on the rug at my feet. Water streamed off him, puddling around me. But he didn't move except for the rising and falling of his ribs as he breathed. I covered him with a towel and took his temperature—100.5. He was getting warmer. I fed him some more colostrum and refilled the sink with warm, clean water. I could almost sleep, propped against the kitchen counter, warming the lamb. At least I relaxed some. It was easier to be doing something when I had a sick lamb.

One hour and two changes of water later, he lifted his head and started to struggle in the sink. I pulled him out and took his temperature—103 degrees. I rubbed him down, fed him two more ounces of colostrum, and laid him by the woodstove to warm. It was time for me to check the ewes in the barn again.

IF CATASTROPHES WOULD happen all by themselves, they might be manageable. But while I was trying to revive 52, Polar Bear was out in the barn having troubles of her own. Polar Bear was huge, she had been for weeks. She normally has twins, so the size was not surprising. But the amount of trouble she was having with this birth was unusual. Polar Bear had obviously been in labor the last time I checked the ewes. She was pawing the straw and straining, her nose tipped up, mouth open, panting. I expected to find new babies on this trip to the barn.

No new babies, just Polar Bear, pawing the straw and straining. Three hours was a long time for a four-year-old ewe to labor over twins. I checked the straw around her to see if her water had broken. The straw was so full of manure and urine this far into lambing that I couldn't tell.

I maneuvered Polar Bear into a corner of the barn. Then I washed my hands (and arms) and knelt beside her. "It's okay," I said. "I'm going to see if I can tell what's going on in here." I squeezed cold lubricating jelly onto my right hand and slid it into Polar Bear's vagina.

Nose. Big nose. I worked my hand back along the lamb's head. The nose continued forever. This was a huge lamb. No wonder Polar Bear was having a hard time. Finally my fingers curved around the side of the lamb's jaw, and I felt hooves. There was no room for my hands to explore further. I hoped that both these hooves were attached to the same lamb and that it was the lamb whose nose was almost ready to deliver. I pressed the lamb's hoof between two fingers and pulled. The hoof slid forward. I pulled again. Then I hooked my fingers around the curve of the lamb's jaw and pulled.

Polar Bear was grunting louder than I had ever heard in a sheep. I was afraid I was hurting her. But this lamb was not coming out on its own, so I had to help. I pulled a little on the hoof again. Then on the curve of the jaw. Finally I slid the fingers of my left hand into Polar Bear's rectum and pulled forward on the ridge of the lamb's forehead, which I could easily feel through the thin tissue separating the two channels. The lamb's nose appeared, followed closely by two little white hooves. I grabbed the hooves and pulled out and down.

Slowly, slowly, the lamb eased out of his mother's uterus. I laid him on the straw and wiped the membrane from his face. He gasped a few times and then began breathing strongly. Lying stretched on the straw, the lamb seemed almost as long as his mother's body. His head and chest were the largest I'd ever seen.

Polar Bear clambered to her feet and began cleaning her baby, a good mother in spite of her tiredness. I rubbed the lamb down, trimmed his umbilical cord, and dipped it in iodine. Then I built a jug around Polar Bear and the lamb and hung up a heat lamp. When I left Polar Bear, her lamb was nursing, and there was no sign yet of a twin.

LIKE POLAR BEAR, I had to continue my job, no matter how tired I was. I tried to get 53 to nurse. I pushed him against his mother's udder and held him in place with my knees. Then I held his mouth open and tried to stuff a nipple into it with my finger. He shut his mouth on my finger, and the nipple squirted out the side. I tried again, keeping my finger outside the lamb's mouth. This time the lamb didn't even close his mouth. He just stood there with his mouth open, his mother's nipple lying on his tongue. Discouraged, I gave him some more colostrum and took his temperature. Normal. Thank goodness!

52's temperature was also normal when I checked it, and the warmth of the woodstove had dried him. I fed him one more bottle of colostrum and carried him out to the barn. I rejugged him with Sprinkle and his brother, 53.

I checked Polar Bear again. No new lambs, but her

placenta was pooled in the corner of the jug. No more lambs for her this year. Out of curiosity, I scooped up the lamb and hung it in the weighing bucket. Sixteen pounds! No wonder Polar Bear had had such a hard time. Her lamb was 10 percent of her normal weight.

Polar Bear's baby, number 69, thrived. Sprinkle's babies didn't. By the time they were a week old, both 52 and 53 had diarrhea, yellow feces staining their hind legs. We started feeding them an electrolyte solution instead of milk. They looked cold, standing all hunched up again. I put them back in a jug and turned on the heat lamp.

The next morning, 53 was lying on the straw with his head turned back along the side of his body and a stiff neck. I rushed him into the house and took his temperature. Ninety-six degrees. I floated him in the sink. Two hours later, his temperature was back to normal. But he wouldn't suck on a bottle. I held him in my lap and slipped the stomach tube down his throat.

I was beyond fear now. I just did the things that had to be done, whether I knew how to do them or not. The last time I used the stomach tube on a lamb, I felt panic inside me, ready to overwhelm me the minute I relaxed my guard. This time, there was no room for panic. I was too intent or too determined or too tired.

I filled a 60-cc syringe with electrolyte solution and forced it into the tube running to 53's stomach. He didn't cough or gasp or die. The food had gone to his stomach, not his lungs.

I laid 53 on the floor by the woodstove and then went to the barn to check on the lambs and ewes. Everyone looked fine except for 52, who was shivering under the heat lamp. I turned off the lamp and tucked him under my arm. Might as well have two lambs in the house as one.

I filled the sink and floated 52 in the warm water.

His temperature wasn't as low as 53's, but I wasn't taking any chances. Ninety minutes later his temperature was normal, and he was thrashing around in the sink.

Now I had two lambs in the living room. I fed them both by bottle. They were obviously feeling better, they ran up to me, eager to nurse. When 52 was dry, I moved them both to a corner of the kitchen. I set table leaves around them as barriers and hung a heat lamp from my roller towel rack. Even I, with my elastic notions on cleanliness, couldn't have lambs with diarrhea on the living room carpet. But my kitchen was a disaster!

The sink was full of dirty water. The counters were covered with dirty dishes. The floor was covered with water, muddy footprints, and yellow-stained towels.

But I had saved two lambs. The feelings of joy and accomplishment were intense. Those feeling were what made lambing so exhilarating, that feeling of power when I did something well.

Six hours later the joy and exhilaration had all drained away. 53 was shivering again. I lowered the heat lamp even further and turned the thermostat in the house to eighty degrees. He wouldn't nurse on the bottle, so we began gavage feedings again. And the yellow diarrhea was still streaming down their legs.

At 10 P.M. I fed them both again. They nursed well. Then 53 stopped breathing. "Dave!" I shouted. "He's dead. He can't be dead. He just nursed."

Dave picked 53 up and held him in his lap. "His heart is still beating," he said. Dave held the little white head in his hand. Then he pressed his lips to the lamb's nose and blew in. 53's ribs moved. Dave blew again. The ribs expanded again. Dave breathed again for the lamb. Then he stopped.

"His heart stopped," Dave said. "I'm sorry, Joanie."

I took the lamb's body out of Dave's lap. "He seemed better. He nursed on the bottle," I said. "Why did he die?" I rubbed my cheek across his little white head. These were the lambs that I wasn't going to bond to. With six bottle lambs, I shouldn't have been able to tell them apart. It wasn't supposed to hurt so much. But I knew 53 and 52. They were important to me. Their lives and deaths mattered.

The ground was too hard, and we were too tired, to dig a grave. I wrapped 53 in a plastic bag and set him in the garbage can with the other lambs who had died this year. Some day they would be fertilizer for the grass and flowers and trees that grew over the dump. Some day I would forget them. Some day.

Dave left for his week at the hospital. 52 was not doing well. Dr. Weckwerth suggested I change electrolytes to a gel that would definitely stop the diarrhea. I should have called him earlier. Maybe I could have saved 53 if I could have stopped his diarrhea. I should have known that there were different electrolytes for different situations.

By evening I had doubts that I could save 52. His breathing was labored. I found him standing in the corner of the kitchen with the underside of his chin pressed against the wall, his face pointing up. He walked almost as if he were blind.

The vets had gone home, it was after 5 P.M. I got out my books and carefully reread the medical section on lambs. Only one disease listed yellow watery diarrhea: *Clostridium perfringens* type B. I'd never heard of it before. We vaccinate for types C and D, but I'd never heard of type B.

I called the vet on call. "It's not very common," Dr. Hexum said. "But I have some antiserum on hand."

"My books say that the antiserum usually doesn't help," I said. "Is that true?"

"Yes," he agreed. "But sometimes if you catch it early enough, you can save the lamb."

"I'll come to your house to pick it up," I said.

"No." His voice was kind. "I have to go to town, I'll leave it in your mailbox in about an hour."

While I waited, I warmed 52 in the sink again. His neck was stiff. Dr. Hexum hadn't been encouraging. I didn't have much hope for the antiserum; 52 had been sick for far too long. If a lamb couldn't regulate his own body temperature under a heat lamp in a warm house, something was seriously wrong with his body besides diarrhea.

Before Amber and Laurel headed up to bed, I told them that 52 would probably die. They'd both been feeding the bottle lambs—Laurel in the morning, and Amber after school. They knew all six lambs by looks and personality. They had grieved at 53's death and had been worrying about 52 all day with me.

Laurel went right to the lamb. She cuddled him, patting his head and talking to him. Then she started to cry. We went upstairs, Laurel and I, and talked on her bed.

"Why does he have to die?"

"Because he is very sick, and I don't know how to make him better."

"Doesn't the vet?"

"No, punkin. We don't know as much about sheep as about people. And maybe even a person would die from this disease."

"I wish people and animals didn't die."

"So do I, punkin. So do I." I held Laurel until her tears dried, until her body relaxed into sleep. Then I went to find Amber.

Amber had taken my bald statement about 52 with stony-faced silence. Her first bottle lamb, Dusty, had died four years earlier. This was the first year she had been able to force herself into the lambing barn again. This year, her grief at Dusty's death was far enough away so that she could allow herself to care about the lambs. And this year, she was being hurt again.

Amber generally dealt with grief by retreating into herself, displaying no emotion. I expected to find her in her room trying to read.

I found her in the kitchen holding 52 in her lap, eyes closed, tears glistening on her cheeks. My chest tightened with love and pride. Love that she cared so much for these little lambs, and pride that she could set aside her own pain to give comfort to a dying lamb. I sat down beside her and put my arm around her, pulling her close to my body.

"You feel really bad about this lamb," I said. Amber nodded, resting her head on my shoulder.

"Are you angry at me for letting him die?"

"It's not your fault," Amber said. "Sometimes lambs just die."

I was glad Amber believed that. She had felt guilt over Dusty's death for a long time.

Amber believed it. Laurel believed it. Why couldn't I believe it? Why couldn't I accept that sometimes lambs just die, and let them go? Why did I tear myself up inside agonizing over each sick animal?

If I knew more about sheep, they wouldn't die. If I watched them more closely, they wouldn't die. If there were two of me instead of just one or thirty hours in a day instead of twenty-four, then maybe I could catch every sick lamb just as it became sick. Maybe I could help every ewe that had a hard labor.

But I was only one person, and there were only twenty-four hours in a day. My feelings of grief and inadequacy when things went wrong were the down side of lambing. The down side could be a very long way down.

52's breathing was becoming very irregular, and his body began to twitch. I didn't want Amber to watch him die. "It's time for bed, love," I told her. "I'm going out to get the medicine the vet left. Why don't you climb into bed and read for a while?" I hugged her. "I love you."

Amber laid the lamb on the floor. She stroked its body one last time and got slowly to her feet. "I love you, too, Mommy. Good night."

"Good night, princess. I'll be right back." Amber dragged up to bed. I shrugged into my parka and boots, put the flashlight in my pocket, and trudged up the driveway.

Ten steps from the door, I was in complete darkness. No moon. No stars. The sky overhead was black. The house lights weren't even reflected from the clouds or the snow. I turned on the flashlight. A tunnel of light advanced before me up the driveway, bouncing back off snowdrifts when I veered toward the edges and swallowed up in darkness when I was walking straight up the drive.

The vial of antiserum was in the mailbox. I hurried back to the house, staggering from snowbank to snowbank across the driveway as I tried to read the directions and keep to the center of the driveway at the same time.

Inside the house, I dropped my jacket on the floor and slipped out of my boots. 52 was still alive. I gave him 25cc of antiserum subcutaneously, a huge injection for such a tiny lamb. Then I fed him and sat down beside him to keep my vigil. His breathing was very ragged, and the muscle twitches kept getting worse.

At 2 A.M. I called Dave. "52 is dying. How can I put him to sleep?"

"Tell me what you see," Dave said.

"I can't keep his temperature up. His breathing is real uneven. His nose is sort of white instead of pink. And his body keeps twitching." My voice broke. "I gave him the antiserum five hours ago, but he just keeps getting worse. I don't want him to suffer anymore."

"Well, it's real bad that he can't regulate his own temperature," Dave agreed. "The breathing and the twitching sound bad, too. I think you're right, he's dying." Dave was quiet for a minute. "I think there is some Demerol in my drug kit. Try giving him that. He should fall asleep and then die very easily." His voice softened. "Call me if you need me."

I ground the Demerol to a powder and mixed it with 50cc of the electrolyte solution. Then I slipped the feeding tube down 52's throat and squirted the solution down the tube.

The Demerol worked fast. Within thirty minutes, 52's body was relaxing. The twitches stopped. His breathing eased. Then he started to drool. He was obviously in deep sleep and no longer feeling pain. I laid him down under the heat lamp. He didn't need me anymore. I didn't need to be with him. He would sleep until he died and not be frightened or hurt.

I pulled on my coveralls and boots to check the ewes. Everyone seemed happy. By now it was almost 3:30 A.M. I staggered back to the house, dropped my coveralls to the floor, and climbed into bed, clothes and all.

The clock radio went on at seven o'clock. The kids woke me at seven-thirty. "Did 52 die?" they asked, afraid to go downstairs without knowing the answer.

"I don't know," I told them. "I gave him some medicine last night that would help him die." Seeing their puzzled looks, I hurried on. "He was getting sicker and sicker. The medicine the vet brought wasn't helping." I hugged Laurel and Amber to me. "So Daddy and I figured out how to give him some medicine that would make him stop hurting and let him die."

"How?" Laurel asked.

"The medicine relaxed his muscles, so that he could breathe easier and his muscles weren't twitching," I explained. "But if you relax muscles enough, the muscles in the heart and around the lungs stop working. That's what I did for 52. I gave him enough relaxing medicine so that the muscles would all relax. He wasn't hurting anymore. Then gradually he stopped breathing, and his heart stopped beating, and he was dead." They looked at me with blank white faces. "I didn't want him to die. But he was dying. And he was hurting. That was the only way that I could help him anymore. Do you understand?"

Both girls nodded and hugged me. We all had tears in our eyes. "Hey, we'd better get going, the bus comes in half an hour." Amber and Laurel went to dress. I went downstairs to remove 52.

52 was standing up, looking toward the stairs.

"Amber! Laurel!" I shouted. "He's alive!"

Both kids clattered downstairs and hugged the lamb. While they fixed and ate their breakfasts, they plied me with questions. "Why is he still alive?"

"I don't know."

"Does that mean he's getting well?"

"I don't know."

"Can we feed him with the bottle?"

"I don't know; we can try." 52 nursed on the bottle hungrily. He was so improved. No muscle tremors, no problem breathing, no diarrhea. Maybe he would live.

James Herriot once put a ewe to sleep, only to have it recover several days later. Maybe I had done the same thing.

The girls kissed the lamb and me goodbye and hurried up the driveway to the bus stop. I went out to the barn to check the ewes. Everybody was fine. When I returned to the house, I fed 52 again with the bottle. Then I lay down beside his pen to nap.

When I woke up at noon, lamb number 52 was dead.

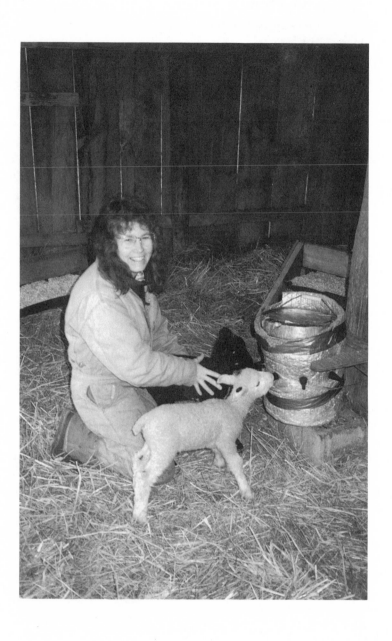

Spirit

Lambs 52 and 53 had died. But Polar Bear's lamb number 69 grew rapidly. Soon he was old enough to get some of his food from the hay feeders that the ewes ate from. He mobbed the feeders with the other lambs, climbing through the feeding holes and eating from the inside out. When we added new hay to the feeders, the lambs squirted out through the feeding holes or jumped over the top bar of the feeder to get away from the thrown bales of hay. Sometimes they jumped into and out of the feeders just for the joy of jumping.

On a late-afternoon trip to the barn, I found 69 hanging from the hay feeder, his hind feet tangled in the bars of the feeder, his front feet on the ground. One of his hind feet was twisted at a ninety-degree angle to the rest of his leg. He was bleeding.

Supporting his body under my left arm, I untangled his legs from the feeder. I carried him toward the house, running. About halfway there, I remembered that I shouldn't let his broken leg dangle, so I rested it on my arm.

"Dave," I said as I walked in the door, "I have a problem here."

We found the break in the main bones of the upper

part of his foot. Then we called the vet. Everyone was out on emergencies, so we splinted it ourselves. Dave cut a piece of plywood to match the angle of his other leg, and we wrapped it to his leg with strips of sheet. Laurel helped by holding the sheet strips. Amber finished feeding the bottle lambs.

"Is he going to die?" they asked.

"Not if I can help it!"

"No," said Dave. "Lambs don't die from broken legs."

About three hours later, the vet on call finally got home. He okayed what we'd done, prescribed 2cc penicillin intramuscularly, and told us to bring the lamb in the next day for a tetanus shot.

So we again had a lamb in the kitchen, and it would be really hard not to bond with this one. We had just castrated him, so we couldn't keep him for breeding stock. We certainly didn't need extraneous male lambs in our flock.

"We can't keep him," I warned the kids. "So don't get attached."

He didn't nurse well on the bottle, drinking maybe one ounce four or five times all night. For a three-week-old lamb, that wasn't much milk. I worried that by the time we got him back out in the pasture, Polar Bear wouldn't accept him. What's more, he hadn't urinated since we found him. Dehydration might become a real problem.

Dr. Weckwerth gave him a tetanus shot and created an enormous walking splint out of white tape and wire. Number 69 still wouldn't walk. When I set him on four feet, he'd only stand on the tip of his right hind foot, the one that wasn't broken.

And he still wouldn't drink much milk from a bottle. I laid him back down and forced some milk into him by squeezing the bottle. We weighed him—twenty-five pounds. We gave him two baby aspirin.

I stood him on his feet again. The casted leg splayed out to his side, unable to support weight. He still rested on the tip of his right hind foot. "I don't think that foot is broken," Dave said, carefully feeling it. "But the tendon might be bruised and sore. Let's splint that one, too."

Number 69's second splint was obviously home-made, a strip of sheet metal strapped to his leg with duct tape (an all-purpose farm tool). Amazingly, with both hind legs splinted, he stood correctly.

Finally, he peed. I took him outside and set him down in the frozen pasture. He immediately started bleating and staggering across the ground, searching for his mother. Number 69 sniffed and rejected three white ewes before he found Polar Bear. She was interested in him, sniffed him thoroughly, but wouldn't let him nurse. When she walked away, he fell.

He looked so pathetic, two splinted legs sprawled on the ground, trying to get up and get to his mother. We caught Polar Bear and number 69 and rejugged them. The next time I checked in the barn, he was nursing. Twelve hours later we let them out of the jug. Number 69 was slow, but when Polar Bear stopped walking, he caught up and nursed.

One week later I walked out the barn door to be engulfed by a flock of running lambs. They were circling the barn, lap after lap. At the back of the pack, last but still in the running, came number 69. His splinted legs threw off his gait, but nothing threw off his spirit.

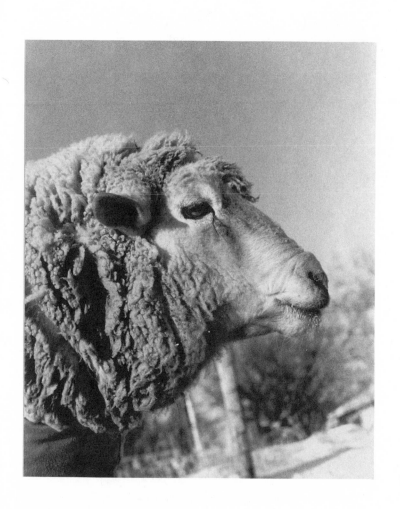

To Market, to Market

By September, our pastures were brown and dry. The water hoses froze most nights. It was time to begin feeding hay. Time to separate the ewes into breeding groups, each with their own ram. Three rams, three breeding groups, three pastures to which I had to haul hay and water.

I didn't want to haul hay and water for lambs that were going to be sold. So we were taking all the extra lambs to market—both the ewe lambs that I didn't want in the flock and the ram lambs. All the ram lambs, even number 69.

Number 69 had recovered very well from his broken bones. By the end of June, when we took the splints off, he could run as fast as any of the other lambs. In late September, I couldn't even tell which lamb he was.

Our marketing had changed over the years to a technique that caused me less pain. We only named the lambs we were adding to the flock, and we castrated the rams so there was no possibility of keeping them. And we sold the lambs by the truckload to the stockyard in West Fargo. By the time we had wrestled fourteen lambs into the back of the pickup, we were so tired and frustrated that we hated them all. Selling them was no longer painful.

The last lamb onto the truck in our second load was 69. I noticed his green ear tag with the number 69 scrawled across it when Dave pushed him up the ramp to me. I shoved him into the pickup and slammed the gate shut. I looked number 69 over as I leaned against the truck, panting. He was taller than the other lambs and seemed just as heavy. He had grown well, even with two broken legs.

Dave and I climbed into the cab and began the ninety-minute drive to the stockyards. I thought about number 69. I remembered how he had looked hanging from the feeder, and how frightened I had been carrying him to the house. I remembered his determined staggers across the barnyard in pursuit of his mother. In my mind I could see him racing around the barn, white splinted legs awkward but fast as he rounded the corner neck and neck with the other lambs, holding his own with no problem.

I had kept him alive for four extra months. Really, he had kept himself alive. All I had done was make the decision not to kill a badly injured lamb. It hadn't even occurred to me to kill him. My job was keeping lambs alive.

So here I was, four months later, selling lambs to the stockyard, which would sell them to feeder operations to be fattened for slaughter.

Usually the contradiction there didn't bother me anymore. But with number 69 in the truck, the lambs had all reverted to cute little animals with personalities. I was no longer selling fourteen trouble-making, stubborn pains in the neck. These were fourteen cuddly white lambs, some of whom I had coaxed into life. All of whom I'd watched and worried over since March.

"Why are we doing this?" I asked Dave.

"You don't want to haul water and hay for forty-two extra sheep," he said.

A scruffy twenty-five-year-old red pickup was a strange setting for a discussion about ethics.

"No, I mean why are we raising animals for slaughter?" I felt my face flushing and heard a thickness in my voice.

Dave obviously heard it, too. His answer was matter-of-fact. "We raise sheep because it is environmentally the best way to treat our land."

"We could let it go to grasses and trees naturally," I answered.

"Only a rich person can afford to let land lie fallow."

"Do you mean," I asked acidly, "that we kill lambs so that no one will know that you earn as much money as the next physician?"

"The sheep convert grass, a poor protein source, to meat, a good protein source," Dave said. "We're doing a good thing, Joanie. We're producing good protein off of marginal land. It means that we don't have to till the fields every year, so we have less erosion. We don't have to use as much fertilizer or pesticide."

"You care more about the land than the sheep!" I said angrily.

"The sheep are part of the land," Dave explained. "But if you're asking me if the sheep have a right to live, I don't know."

"If I believe that the sheep have a right to live, then I can't let extra sheep be born," I said. "So I guess that is what I'm asking."

"Joanie," Dave said patiently, "we give them good, if short, lives. They have plenty of food and water. They are protected from predators and disease. You leave them with their mothers until they go to market. They are happy."

"I feel like I'm betraying them," I said. Tears pooled in my eyes. "The stockyards are big and scary. And who knows what the feeder lots are like? They always look crowded, hot, and filthy." I wiped my cheeks angrily. "I shouldn't be doing that to the lambs."

"So what are your alternatives?" Dave asked.

"Amundson Meats seems humane. They keep the animals in a cool, dark barn in stalls bedded with straw. They kill them quickly." I wiped my eyes again and sniffed. "Maybe I should try to sell more freezer lambs. At least then I would know what happens to them."

"It would mean a lot more work for you," Dave said.

"I know," I answered. "And I hate the marketing part. But maybe it's my responsibility."

Tears drying on my cheeks, I thought about my responsibilities. Farming, like mothering, is a very self-propelled job. Only my conscience tells me what to do. My conscience tells me to make a nutritious dinner for the family and to feed the sheep good hay. My conscience forces me to make dental appointments and to learn to castrate lambs. My conscience encourages me to discipline the kids when they need it, even when I don't want to. And now my conscience was encouraging me to learn another disagreeable part of farming—marketing.

To be the best shepherdess I can, perhaps I must not relinquish control until the lamb is killed.

"What would we have to do to sell more freezer lambs?" I asked Dave.

"Well," he answered, "you'd have to advertise so that people would know you had a product to sell."

"I'd have to find out how many lambs Amundson's could handle at a time, and what the best time of year was for him."

"Probably you should find out about the legality of selling freezer meat if you're going to expand," Dave continued.

"And I should buy a new ram. I've read that Texel rams produce leaner lambs, and that their offspring grow faster. I could use him to produce freezer lambs and one of my fleece rams to produce lambs with beautiful fleeces, which I could add to my flock."

"You could maybe sell more breeding stock," said Dave. "That way you'd send fewer lambs to market."

"I'd have to do advertising for that, too," I said. "But I think it would be worth it."

Excitement had replaced my tears. The scruffy red pickup had been a good place for a philosophical discussion, after all. If everything worked out, we would be heading in a new, more compassionate direction with our sheep.

We backed up to the loading ramp at the stockyards. I caught lamb number 69 first. I pressed my face against his soft woolly body. "I'm sorry," I said. "I'll try hard not to do this again. Thank you. Thank you for your life."

I pulled number 69 down the ramp, and the other thirteen lambs followed him. There was no escape for these castrated ram lambs. They couldn't be used as breeding stock. They were too big to be bought for pets. It was too late in the season for anyone to need lawn mowers.

"Thank you," I said as I closed and locked the gate behind them. "Thank you."

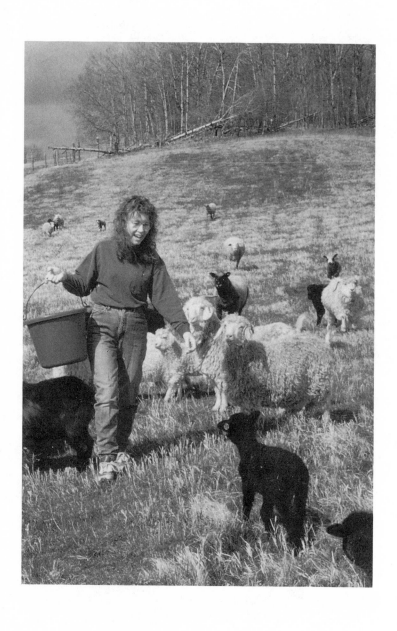

Shepherdess!

even years ago I bought four sheep as pets. They were the beginning of my search for respect and income in the real world.

I carried a picture of myself as a shepherdess for all that time: dressed in tight blue jeans, shiny black boots, a rose-and-blue plaid shirt, and a blue down vest, with rose nail polish on my beautifully manicured nails and exquisite makeup on a face framed by honey-brown curls.

I have no idea where the image came from, certainly no farming reality I've ever seen. Reality is manure-covered boots, loose, ragged jeans, and yesterday's dirty T-shirt, all covered by bulky, filthy brown coveralls. Reality is ragged fingernails caked with dirt, smears of dirt on my face, and my hair scraped back under a scarf.

My dreams and reality did cross once, however. The local newspaper came to take photographs this last year during shearing. I dressed for shearing in tight new jeans, shiny black rubber barn boots (freshly washed for the occasion), a rose-and-blue plaid shirt, and my blue down vest. I made up my face and left my honey-brown hair curling around my face. It was too cold to work without gloves, so I didn't bother to polish my nails.

It was also too cold to work without long underwear. Before we sheared the first ewe, I went back to the

153

house to put on long underwear. I didn't look quite as svelte, but I felt much warmer.

By the time the *Press* photographer arrived, I had manure on my boots and stains on the knees of my new, tight jeans. My hair was driving me crazy. Every time I leaned forward to give a shot, my honey-brown curls fell in front of my face and obscured my view. I tied my hair back with a piece of baling twine. When the photographer left, I put on my coveralls.

The *Press* was doing an article on *me*, a woman who raised sheep so that she would have wool to spin. But it wasn't me the shepherdess who intrigued them, it was me the spinner.

The amazing thing about the interview was how much I talked. I spoke enthusiastically about sheep characteristics and fleece characteristics. The reporter encouraged me. I pointed out the advantages of manure and doing pelvic exams. The reporter was appalled. I described pulling lambs out of ewes and castrating rams. The reporter was horrified. I discussed breeding for knitting wool and multiple births. The reporter was bored. Finally I ran out of steam, and he escaped. It had been a wonderful interview! I was surprised at how much knowledge I had gathered over seven years. I loved talking about the sheep, loved being an expert.

Of course, it was easy being an expert in front of a city-bred newspaper reporter. I played expert again several weeks later when I sold Solomon to a man who had read the article. He was just starting in sheep and wanted to make lots of money from sheep that would have twins and triplets. I explained about Finn sheep and multiple births. Solomon was a Finn-Lincoln cross, perfect for him. Then he asked me how much I earned per sheep per year.

My fleece sales were fantastic! Selling to handspinners by mail, I could earn four to eight times the market price on wool. But I hadn't figured out the best way to sell the rest of my crop.

The sheep books and agricultural extension handouts all mentioned one hundred dollars per ewe per year. My upper limit had been considerably lower than the books suggested, and for God knows how many hours of labor. Not just work, labor. Typing is work, dishwashing is work. Raising sheep is labor, where you use your muscles and sweat and grunt. Hard labor.

Dave feels that the labor in and of itself makes the job worthwhile. I don't. Labor is good. Thinking is good. Learning is good. But no one of them is enough if you are only pretending you are earning a living at it. After all, who in their right mind would cut off tails, explore uteruses, and shovel manure for about a thousand dollars a year? As my friend Barry mused, "I wonder if the IRS would believe I have one hundred dependents?"

I've gained more than knowledge about sheep. I now have a new way of looking at life, and at death. The sheep have taken me in other, unanticipated directions. I've begun to write about the sheep, and people read what I write and sometimes even pay me to write it. I've also come to respect farmers immensely and to mourn their dying life-style. A lot of them are having a hard time earning a living at farming.

My income should go up this year. I bought a new terminal sire, a ram used to father rams for the slaughter market. His lambs will gain weight much faster than my Finn cross lambs. When you double the size of the lamb, you double your income. I'm also going to look into specialty markets, such as organic lamb and lamb by mail.

THAT IS, I'll do these things if I continue with the sheep. After seven years, it's really time to assess what I'm doing, why I'm doing it, and what the results are.

I set out to become an expert, craving all those things that "expert" implies: recognition, acceptance, respect, income, and self-confidence. And it does seem like everyone in town knows who I am, thanks to the newspaper article. But the people who really matter, my family and friends, always knew who I was, sometimes better than I did.

I wanted acceptance in our community. Well, our acceptance began the very day we drove into town in a beat-up red pickup truck loaded with our furniture. "You wouldn't have fit in," said Howard, "if you'd begun farming with a new four-wheel-drive pickup. Your old red pickup showed you were real people." The town's acceptance of me grew as I volunteered with Camp Fire, the school, and our church. And this acceptance had nothing to do with my expertise. It was based on me the person, not me the shepherdess.

This last winter I was asked to join Rotary as a shepherdess. I was honored; it signified the ultimate confirmation of my title in our rural community. So no one was more surprised than I was when I declined. But I realized then that being a Rotarian or a Sunday school teacher or a successful shepherdess doesn't bring one respect. Knowing deep inside yourself what kind of a person you are, liking that person, and being proud of that person bring the only kind of respect that is worth having: self-respect.

I SET OUT to become a shepherdess without knowing what was involved, and I made plenty of mistakes. But after seven years, I can look at my accomplishments with some satisfaction.

Our farm is healthier now than it was when we bought it. It has more nitrogen and organic matter in the soil. There's more topsoil on the hills and lower levels of pesticides in the valleys. We've planted trees to catch the snow for moisture, and we've stopped planting crops in the sloughs. We've been good stewards for our land.

I have learned to keep my sheep healthy. They are raised humanely and happily. They don't smile much, but the lambs gambol all the time, and the ewes gambol when the weather turns cool. Gamboling is happiness in motion. The lambs are weaned by their mothers when the time is right. They have plenty of food and water and are protected from predators and stress.

I have determined the optimum end products in both wool and meat and am learning to breed for those goals. Since a ewe's fleece doesn't sell for enough money to pay for her yearly upkeep, her lambs must be sold for meat. I try to do that in the best way possible. I keep them at home with their flock until it is time for them to die. They have a short trip to the slaughterhouse, where they are killed cleanly and quickly.

If I can't sell them for meat, I can't allow them to be born. Being a shepherdess is a job, not a charity. To live, they have to die. I must ensure that their deaths, as well as their lives, are good.

I no longer spend most of lambing season frantically paging through sheep books. I solve most of the problems myself or with Dave's help. If I'm not sure of something, I call the veterinarians, unselfconsciously. "I think I'm giving the lambs the wrong antibiotic," I say over the phone. "Would something else be better?"

I can turn to other farmers for help and reassurance. "Were the rains in March hard on your stock?" I ask an old dairy farmer. "I lost six lambs and three ewes."

"If you can't take an animal dying," he says looking off at his cows, "you can't be a farmer."

So there is the crucial question. Can I be a farmer? Do I want to be a farmer? Part of being a farmer is accepting the deaths of your animals. Another part is accepting the hard work and the low pay. Part of being a farmer is hearing your daughter ask, "Why don't you work, Mommy?" and hearing an urban cousin say "Ugh! That's all right. You don't have to tell me about lambing."

Part of being a farmer is the final admission that I am no longer a biochemist. I haven't been one for years, of course, but it was the last job listed on my résumé. Now I write "shepherdess" on forms that ask my occupation. I answer "shepherdess" when people ask me what I do.

Was becoming a mother and a shepherdess a good trade for my biochemistry? I don't know. I don't talk with physicians, biochemists, and geneticists at dinner parties anymore. Now I talk with teachers, artists, mothers, volunteers, bus drivers, businessmen, and other shepherds. The conversations range much further and perhaps are closer to reality than they were when I mostly talked biochemistry.

I do miss being part of an intellectual elite at a research institution. But if I were still a biochemist, I wouldn't have seen my moon-cast shadow cross the barnyard in front of me at 3 A.M. on a still March night. I wouldn't shiver at the coyote howls piercing the dusk when the lambs are small. I wouldn't watch a great blue heron sweeping across the April sky. I wouldn't know the rush of power that comes with saving a lamb. I wouldn't know the tearing grief that accompanies losing a ewe.

The personal costs of being a shepherdess are much higher than I imagined—exhaustion, anguish, depression. Is it worth it?

Well, the sheep are all bred this year. It's my responsibility to get them through this lambing. Then we'll see. Then I'll make a decision. But for now, shepherdesses don't shirk their responsibilities.

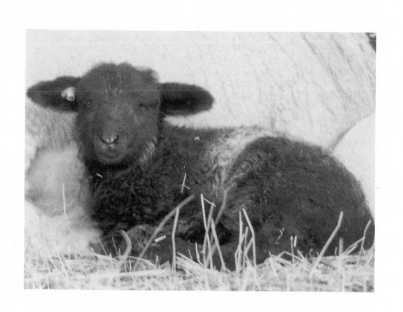

Epilogue

Something was wrong with Brownie. Other than the fact that she looked like a beached whale, I mean. I had found her alone in the barn twice, just lying there. She didn't come out for corn or for the new hay.

"Come on, Brownie, old girl. You have to get up." At 6 A.M. and 9 A.M. she lumbered to her feet at my urging and moved out of the barn. At noon, she was lying in the pasture in the warm sunshine, and I couldn't budge her.

I interrupted Dave's studying. "She's definitely down and I can't move her," I explained. "I think she might have pregnancy toxemia. But I can't hold her nose and hold a keto stick in the appropriate place to collect urine at the same time."

Dave grinned. "I can't imagine why not," he said. "You get the keto sticks while I put on my coveralls."

Back in the pasture, Brownie hadn't moved. "I'll hold her nose and mouth closed so she can't breathe," I said. "You hold the keto stick under the urine stream." Dave looked at me quizzically. "Not being able to breathe is supposed to make them pee," I explained.

"No," Dave said, "I just don't know where to hold the stick."

"Back there under her vulva." I put my hands around

Brownie's mouth and nose, pressing tight. "When the urine comes out, you'll know."

Brownie lay there calmly for the longest time. Finally, she started to struggle, wrenching her head back and forth, trying to pull it out of my tiring hands. "I can't hold on much longer," I gasped.

"There!" Dave shouted, just as Brownie pulled her head out of my hands. "Got it."

"Count fifteen seconds," I said, "then compare the color on the stick with the color on the chart."

Fifteen seconds later Dave looked up. "She has ketosis," he said. "Let's get her into the barn, and then we'll call the vet." Dave was strong enough to hoist Brownie to her feet. Then we pushed and pulled her down the hill and into the corner of the barn where Nutmeg had lived for four weeks last winter. Dave hung a light and set up panels to separate Brownie from the rest of the sheep.

I called the vet, who wasn't in. Linda, his receptionist, relayed my questions through the radio.

"I have a ewe who's very pregnant but not in labor yet. Her urine is positive for ketones. Should we induce her?" I asked.

"Station to Mobile Three," Linda said. "Joan Ellison wants to induce a ewe."

I understand the difficulties in using a radiophone to communicate, but the shorthand always leaves me feeling like I'm trying to practice medicine without a license.

"Why?" asked the disembodied voice of Mobile Three, whoever that was, over two phone systems.

"Her urine is positive for ketones," Linda answered. "Could we use oxytocin?"

"Is her cervix dilated?" the vet asked. "Has her milk come in yet?"

"Did you hear that?" Linda asked me.

"I'll try to find out," I answered. "I'll call you back."

Dave was cleaning and refilling water buckets when I got back to the barn.

"We have to check to see if her cervix is dilated," I said.

"You can do it," Dave said.

"But I don't even know what a cervix feels like, much less how to tell how far it's dilated."

"You can do it," he repeated.

I sudsed my hands and arms well in a bucket of forty-degree water from the barn faucet and knelt beside Brownie. I slid my icy, soapy hand into her vagina. Warmth. I felt warmth, softness, and dark. Eyes shut, I explored the inside of my favorite ewe. Nothing slimy or wet-feeling. I couldn't feel any lamb parts at all, no feet, no nose. Nothing but vague lumps and bumps. Some hard and fixed, others soft and flexible.

"In a human," Dave said, "the cervix is the soft shape coming up from the bottom of the vagina. You can move it around, and hopefully feel the opening in it."

I moved my fingers back and forth over the base of Brownie's vagina. There it was! A little half-inch bump of tissue. No opening into it at all. I removed my hand—cold again. Then we tried stripping milk from her udder. Nothing.

The vet was still out when I called, so we talked through the radiophone. "She's not dilated, and no milk," I said. "But she's enormous. She must be really close to lambing."

"Joan is right," the vet said. "She needs to be induced. But we don't use oxytocin in ruminants. The hormones will take twenty-four to thirty-six hours. In the meantime, start giving her propylene glycol orally every twelve hours."

"Thanks," I told Linda. "I'll be right in to pick up the hormones. I have propylene glycol here."

An hour later I felt much better. We had given Brownie her hormones and were fighting the ketosis with propylene glycol and electrolytes in a gavage bag. It was like *déjà vu,* looking down at one of my colored ewes lying in a dark corner of the barn under a gavage bag. If she would just lamb soon, maybe we could save her.

Twenty-four hours later, the sun was gone, the sky was an ugly gray, and Brownie was worse. I called the vet again. He wasn't there.

"My ewe's breathing is deteriorating. She's breathing very shallowly and panting," I told Linda. "I would be more comfortable if the vet stopped in to see her."

"I'll tell him you called," Linda said. "But he has a breech calf in Lake Park." Lake Park! I had no idea our vets covered such a wide territory. He would be a long time coming.

I headed back out to the barn. In the short time I had been on the phone, the wind had come up. Trees were tossing. Clouds of snow blew across the barnyard. We were in for a storm.

Brownie was even worse. Her tongue was hanging out of her mouth, and her belly was bigger than it had been. Much bigger. I washed and lubricated my hand and slipped it into Brownie's vagina. Her cervix was harder and flatter. She was dilating. But she was getting fatter while I watched, and her breathing was even more labored.

I ran back to the house through the worsening storm. The snow was already starting to drift, and visibility was decreasing.

Dave and the girls looked up as I dashed in the door. "What are you doing home from school?" I asked.

"It's a snow day," Amber said. "How's Brownie?"

"She's worse," I said, pulling off my mittens. "Dave, will you please come out and help?"

While Dave pulled on his coveralls, I called the vet again. "This is Joanie Ellison," I said. "She's getting worse fast. Do you know where we are on his list?"

"He's started back from Lake Park," Linda said. "But the roads are really bad. It's going to take him a while."

"Okay, we'll be out in the barn."

The wind tore at us when we stepped out the door. Snow in the air completely hid the massive bulk of the barn. Only the dim glow from a heat lamp guided us across the home pasture.

In her corner, Brownie lay completely on her side, head stretched out, panting. Her belly was huge, and its shape was wrong. Her belly reached almost to her feet, even when she was lying down, and it bulged everywhere, even along her backbone.

"Could she have ruptured her uterus?" I asked.

"She'd be dead by now," Dave said. He laid his fingers high on her belly and tapped them hard with the fingers of his other hand. He moved his hands to the bottom of her abdomen and tapped again. "Do you hear the difference?" he asked.

I nodded.

"I think there's gas in there," Dave said, pointing to the top of Brownie's abdomen.

"The toxemia must be so bad that her digestion isn't working right. She's bloating!" The specter of bloat has terrified me ever since we first got sheep. When sheep bloat, their rumens, or bellies, fill up with gas. If they swell enough, the rumen could compress the lungs, and the sheep would suffocate.

Howard, our farmer friend, has warned me about

165

bloat every year when we pasture the sheep on the alfalfa. "One could lose a lot of sheep to bloat," Howard would say.

And now I was about to lose Brownie to bloat. "What gauge needle should I use?" I asked Dave.

"The biggest we've got."

I rummaged through the barn cupboard as I spoke. "I'm sure there is a sixteen in here." Twenties, twenty-twos, eighteens. There! The little white plastic tube held a sixteen-gauge needle. I scooped up the needle and a bottle of alcohol.

"Pour the alcohol up here where she sounded hollow."

Dave rubbed the alcohol into Brownie's wool. I pushed the needle into her abdomen. Air whooshed out. "Press all around here until the air stops coming out."

We tapped all over Brownie's belly, inserting the needle and releasing gas until we couldn't find any more hollow-sounding areas. Then we sat back on our heels. Brownie's belly was no longer obscenely swollen. Her breathing was much better. Her tongue was back in her mouth, and she wasn't panting.

"I'm going to check her cervix," I said to Dave. "Why don't you call the vet and tell him we're doing okay?"

This time when I slid my hand into Brownie's vagina, I could feel into her cervix. There was definitely a lamb there, waiting to be born.

I washed and dried my hands. Then I pulled on my mittens and hat and walked the home pasture, checking for lost lambs. There were no lamb-sized bumps under the rapidly drifting snow. I returned to the barn and counted ewes. Everyone was there. I pulled the barn doors shut. This was not a good night for the sheep to be outside.

I stripped off my hat and mittens and brushed the

snow off my coveralls. I took the iodine, knife, and two clean towels to Brownie's pen. Just as I settled myself on the floor, Amber and Laurel blew into the barn, bringing swirls of icy wind and snow. They also brought a thermos of coffee and a pocketful of chocolate chip cookies.

"Is Brownie going to be all right?" Amber asked, sitting down beside her pet ewe in the straw.

"I think so," I said. "I'll be a lot happier when she lambs."

"How many lambs do you think she'll have?" Laurel wanted to know. She walked from jug to jug, checking on each lamb.

"There must be at least two in there. She's so big!"

"Do you think we'll have a snow day tomorrow?" Amber asked.

"If the wind keeps blowing, the buses won't be able to get through."

"Good!" both girls shouted. "The driveway is already blown shut," Laurel added.

I laughed. "Maybe you should head back to the house while you can still see to follow your footprints."

"Will you come with us, Mommy?" Laurel asked. "It's scary out there."

"Okay, I need to talk to your dad anyway," I said. "Let's take one last look at everybody."

Laurel and Amber made the round of the jugs, picking up each lamb to make sure they all stretched contentedly. I returned to Brownie. One last pelvic exam before we went into the house.

I lubricated my hand and slid it in the opening to her vagina. There was a nose right there!

"Brownie's lambing!" I shouted. Amber and Laurel rushed over. I moved my fingers around the little nose to the tiny hooves lying under it. I tugged gently on first one hoof and then the other. Encouraged by my tugs, Brownie's baby squeezed out into the pool of light on the barn floor.

With Amber and Laurel watching breathlessly over my shoulder, I ripped the membrane from the lamb's face. Her chest didn't move. I lifted her and dropped her. Nothing. I repeated the motion again. Still no breaths. I gathered the lamb to my chest and raced for the barn door. "Be right back," I shouted. This lamb had to live. I couldn't let one die right in front of Amber's eyes.

The wind caught at me as I stepped out the door. Stinging the exposed skin on my hands and face, blinding me. I slid my hands along the lamb's body to grasp her hind legs. I stepped away from the building and swung. I pulled her back and laid my face against her body. No movement. I swung again. This time when I laid my face against her, I felt her shuddery first breaths.

Relieved, I stepped back into quiet and warmth of the barn. "Is she all right, Mommy?" Laurel asked. "Another one came."

I looked over at the girls and Brownie huddled in a halo of light at the far end of the barn. Amber was rubbing a second black lamb with a towel. "She's fine," I said. "How's that one?"

"She's breathing all by herself," Laurel answered.

I laid the first lamb down beside Laurel. "Why don't you rub her dry?" I said. Then I turned to Amber, who had tears running down her face. "Why are you crying?" I asked.

"I didn't know what to do!" Amber sobbed.

"The lamb looks just great, you must have done the right thing."

"Laurel pulled it out, and I rubbed it with the towel."

"It started breathing all by itself," Laurel interjected, looking up from the little black lamb she was rubbing.

There was a lump in my throat as I looked down at my two girls. I set my foot into a space in the hog panel around Brownie's pen and swung the other leg over.

"Mom!" Laurel shouted. "Here comes another lamb!"

In my rush to join them in the pen, I tripped, sliding my leg further through the opening in the hog panel. "You'll have to catch this one, too, Laurel," I said, struggling to get my foot untangled. "I'm stuck."

Laurel set her lamb beside Brownie's head and then moved behind the big ewe. I caught my balance and pulled my foot out of the hog panel just as Laurel picked Brownie's third baby up from the straw and shook it. "It's breathing!" she announced triumphantly.

I began trimming umbilical cords and dipping them in iodine. "They're all girls!" I said in surprise. "Brownie, you outdid yourself this time! I'm going to start these nursing," I said to Amber and Laurel. "Why don't you check on the lambs and ewes again?" Brownie was so tired that she didn't object when I pushed her leg aside and stripped the milk from her udder without forcing her to stand up. Then I laid the first lamb next to her udder and stuffed a nipple into its mouth. She immediately began to suck. Lambs two and three caught on to nursing just as enthusiastically as the first lamb.

"I think we have everything under control," I said. "Let's go get some dinner."

I turned for one last look at Brownie and her lambs. The golden glow from the heat lamp turned an ordinary farm scene into a magnificent painting of light and dark, life and death, mother love and loving daughters. I sighed with contentment and turned into the blowing snow.

The wind pushed against us as we staggered across the barnyard, searching for holes in our coveralls, finding paths to send snow sneaking in toward our bodies. The house lights glowed warmly in the distance. The barnyard gate was drifted shut. We climbed the stile to get over the fence.

An hour later, I fought my way back across the barnyard. I wanted to check on Brownie and her babies. I wanted to double check all the ewes and lambs.

There was a fourth baby lying in Brownie's pen.

"Oh, Brownie!" I exclaimed. "How could you do this?" The tiny black lamb lay half licked in a corner of the pen. I rested my hand on the body. Cold and slimy. But the ribs moved! This lamb was still alive!

I gathered the little black lamb into my arms and carefully stuffed her into my coveralls, head and all. Then I raced for the house, oblivious to the snow and cold. Thinking only of the tiny half-dead lamb inside my jacket.

"Dave," I gasped as I burst in the doorway, "Brownie had another lamb! Quick, warm some colostrum and find the feeding tube and syringe!" I unzipped my coveralls and brought out the little black lamb. Was she still alive? Yes! Her ribs still moved.

"Amber, get some towels. Laurel, get the dirty dishes out of the sink."

I ran water over my free hand, testing until it was hot enough, but not too hot. Laurel set the plug in the bottom of the sink, and I laid the lamb in the deepening pool of warmth.

"She's so little," Amber said.

"I know. I've never seen such a little lamb," I agreed. "Hope we can keep her alive. She has tried so hard to live. She was ice-cold when I found her."

"Four lambs," Dave said. "I can't believe she had four lambs."

"Brownie was big enough for four lambs," Laurel laughed.

Dave threaded the thin feeder tube down the lamb's throat while I held her head above the water. Then we forced an ounce of warm colostrum into her stomach.

The water in the sink cooled and we refilled it. The lamb lay placidly in my hands. We had just refilled the sink a second time when the lamb started to shiver.

"That's a good sign," Dave said. "I was afraid that her digestion had shut down. Shivering means that her body has enough energy to try to warm itself. She must have digested the colostrum."

We slipped the stomach tube down her throat and gave her another ounce of colostrum. When I pulled the tube out, the lamb jerked her head away from my hand. I drained the water in the sink and began refilling it with warmer water. The lamb floundered out of my hands and struggled to her feet.

"She's standing!" I shouted. "She's going to live."

I set the lamb on the towels and began to dry her off. Water streamed out of her tightly curled wool and puddled around us on the floor.

"She's Brownie's baby," Laurel said. "We could name her after Paul's microwave brownies."

"Yeah," Amber agreed. "We could name her Microwave because she's so small."

"Are you going to keep any lambs?" Dave asked.

From my position beside the lamb I looked up at my family. Was I going to keep any lambs this year? Was I going to keep any sheep? I looked down at the lamb. I thought of Brownie and her three lambs in the barn.

I'd come a long way from Roses' dying baby. A long way from that first cold night of panic in the lambing shed when I first got to know Brownie.

"I think it's too cold for such a little lamb in the barn tonight," I said. "If we're going to keep a lamb in the house, I guess we'll have to keep her forever. Microwave sounds like a great name."